<br>
# Ethics in Art Therapy

*of related interest*

**The Art of Business**
**A Guide to Self-Employment for Creative Arts Therapists**
*Emery Hurst Mikel*
*Foreword by Michael A. Franklin*
ISBN 978 1 84905 950 3
eISBN 978 0 85700 772 8


**Beginning Research in the Arts Therapies**
**A Practical Guide**
*Gary Ansdell and Mercédès Pavlicevic*
ISBN 978 1 85302 885 4
eISBN 978 1 84642 167 9


**Art Therapy Techniques and Applications**
*Susan I. Buchalter*
ISBN 978 1 84905 806 3
eISBN 978 1 84642 961 3

# Ethics
# in Art Therapy

## Challenging Topics for
## a Complex Modality

*Lisa R. Furman*

*Foreword by Deborah Farber*

Jessica Kingsley *Publishers*
London and Philadelphia

Front cover image source: Audrey (2011), title withheld, oil on canvas, 20" x 24".

First published in 2013
by Jessica Kingsley Publishers
116 Pentonville Road
London N1 9JB, UK
and
400 Market Street, Suite 400
Philadelphia, PA 19106, USA

*www.jkp.com*

**Library of Congress Cataloging in Publication Data**
Furman, Lisa R.
Ethics in art therapy : challenging topics for a complex modality / Lisa R. Furman ;
foreword by Deborah
Farber.
pages cm
Includes bibliographical references and index.
ISBN 978-1-84905-938-1 (alk. paper)
1. Art therapy. 2. Art therapy--Moral and ethical aspects. 3. Art therapists--
Professional ethics. I. Title.
RC489.A7F86 2013
174.2'96891656--dc23
2013009200

**British Library Cataloguing in Publication Data**
A CIP catalogue record for this book is available from the British Library

ISBN 978 1 84905 938 1
eISBN 978 0 85700 757 5

Printed and bound in Great Britain by Bell & Bain Ltd, Glasgow

*For my daughter, who inspires me to always seek
a sense of discernment, virtue, and value in my
professional life, and for all of my clients, who remind
me that art therapy is a powerful healing tool.*

# Contents

# List of Figures

# Foreword

It is with great pleasure that I write the foreword for Lisa Furman's book, *Ethics in Art Therapy: Challenging Topics for a Complex Modality*. Professional ethics is an ever evolving construct. This is particularly relevant in contemporary society, given the rapidity with which technological advances occur and the shifting and changing state of American demographics and the economy. In the field of art therapy, the role of the art product in the therapeutic process raises specific considerations in these areas regarding social media, digital imagery, religion and spirituality, and sexuality. It is crucial that graduate students, new professionals, and seasoned clinicians in the creative arts therapies remain current with advances in the field.

Ethics are not static. *Ethics in Art Therapy: Challenging Topics for a Complex Modality* explores these gray areas not generally addressed in professional guidelines and presents concrete examples making theoretical ideas practical. Furman's discussion of how spiritual viewpoints and responses to religious symbolism in art can pose ethical dilemmas which potentially obstruct professional boundaries is of particular importance for art therapists. The use of digital media is an exciting new arena, but haphazard use can breach confidentiality regulations in clinical practice. Lisa Furman guides the reader in how to be ethically responsible in the use of digital communication. Furman applies this ethical decision making process to the theory and practice of art therapy supervision. Utilizing art making in supervision is a complex process, as we can never presume to fully comprehend another person's experience in terms of culture, race, or life circumstance.

Lisa Furman is uniquely qualified to author a book on ethical issues, having developed a series of community lectures on ethics as a faculty member at the School of Visual Arts Master of Professional Studies in Art Therapy Program, which I chair. I have been impressed by her generosity of spirit, her altruism, and her ability to present the subject of ethics in an engaging, sensitive, and on occasion, humorous manner. In addition, Lisa Furman has co-authored (with Michael Fisher, PhD), an ethical principles document for our students and faculty, which has become the cornerstone of our supervision curriculum on ethical guidelines. *Ethics in Art Therapy: Challenging Topics for a Complex Modality* is certainly a fundamental reading that provides an invaluable advancement of art therapy ethics.

*Deborah Farber, MPS, ATR-BC, LCAT*
*Chair, Art Therapy Department*
*School of Visual Arts*

# Acknowledgments

This book would not have been possible without the support and vision of Lisa Clark of Jessica Kingsley Publishers, who first approached me about writing a book on ethics. Infinite gratitude is also expressed to Martha Dorn and Tahlia Furman Cott, for their keen referencing and editing skills which made it possible for me to more wholly focus on writing. The author would also like to express thanks to colleagues and supervisees, including Abbe Miller, Dr. Ragaa Mazen, Dr. Stephen Joy, Evie Lindemann, Rebecca Miller, Stephanie Gorski, Susan Falato, Kim Bella, and Lena Deleo for their invaluable assistance in providing me with ideas for case scenarios, feedback, and kind support along the way. Special thanks to Marilyn Catasus for photographing the artwork of Audrey, and a gracious expression of thanks to Audrey and her husband for sharing the story of her art and life in a way that will no doubt profoundly influence the lives of others. Finally, the author would like to convey deep gratitude to Deborah Farber, Valerie Sereno, and the School of Visual Arts for organizing the community lecture series that inspired this book.

# Disclaimer

This book contains case scenarios that are best understood as conceptualized narratives, containing both fact and fiction, based on collective situations from the author's own experience as well as those reported by supervisees, students and colleagues. Any identifying information that may be related to factual events has been concealed. The case scenarios were created to mimic real life situations in which a practitioner may face an ethical decision. They are intended to be used only for teaching purposes and to stimulate thoughtful discussion of complex ethical topics with the hope that the reader might be able to develop and enhance decision making skills for ethical challenges in daily practice.

# Preface

This book was written based on a series of presentations given as part of the ongoing School of Visual Arts MPS art therapy department community lecture series in New York City from 2009 to 2013. Organized by art therapist Valerie Sereno, the lecture series was conceived by the art therapy department chair, Deborah Farber, as a free educational opportunity to students, alumni, professional art therapists, and interested clinicians in related disciplines in the community. The lecture topics included presentations on the theory and practice of art therapy, including ethical professional practice.

Ethical practice is the backbone of any profession. Most clinical disciplines require participation in a certain amount of ethics instruction in order to maintain licensure or certification, so clinicians are often seeking education in ethics. The topics chosen for the lecture series, and subsequently for this book, were culled from my experience as an internship and post-graduate supervisor and seemed, to me, to be topics of great import, enormous conflict, and immense need amongst my supervisees. Additionally, as an educator, addressing topics of sexuality, physical contact with a client, integrating spirituality into treatment, or informed consent, are most naturally embedded in the internship curriculum, as this is where most incidental learning occurs. My hope is that this book will be a useful addition to ethics curricula in graduate art therapy programs as well as a practical guide for clinicians.

Over the years, I have come to learn that the topics which supervisees save for last, with only moments before the supervision session ends, are the ones that are usually most ethically and clinically challenging. Questions about hugging clients, managing sexual feelings in sessions, or taking digital pictures of client art without permission are usually prefaced with halting appeals for reassurance and guidance. It is in these moments, I believe, when a supervisee expresses a willingness to explore their established ethical values that large-scale learning can occur.

My students and supervisees have come to know me as an instructor who is generally comfortable with the uncomfortable, allowing me to initiate topics of gravity with humor and grace. Once they are comfortable with my style as an educator, they also know that if they ask a question, even one that deals with embarrassing content, they will get an honest answer, without feeling any humiliation in raising the topic. I believe that it is essential to create a comfortable climate in the learning environment, otherwise supervisees will not seek out guidance if they feel that they will be shamed in the process. Avoidance of supervision only leads to covert breaches of ethics with no recourse for growth and change. Nothing is more isolating in a decision making process than feeling as though one has nowhere to turn for counsel.

Further, as an ethics educator, I do not suggest that I am flawless; in fact, I am fairly open about using my own mistakes as examples of learning to help encourage a supportive learning atmosphere. In the process, I also let my supervisees know that I always have the client's needs as foremost in my decision making process, along with motives that are well intended. If nothing else, second only to my unbridled enthusiasm about the healing power of art therapy, a willingness to continue to evolve as a more ethical art therapist while still embracing all of my shortcomings has always been my primary aspiration. I am hoping the reader will feel the same about this book and not be deterred by the solemnity of the topics, or any harsh and unnecessary self appraisal that often inhibits introspective discussions about ethics.

*Note:* When referring to an individual art therapist, gendered pronouns have been alternated by chapter for ease of reading.

# Introduction

## Ethical Decisions in Art Therapy Practice

### The complexities of art therapy practice

Art therapists are often confronted with ethical dilemmas that are unique to the field because of the complicated nature of utilizing imagery and art materials in clinical practice (Green 2012; Hinz 2011; Moon 2006). The content of artwork is generally regarded as a form of communication, a kind of symbolic language that is afforded the same protection as verbal content in treatment (Hammond and Gantt 1998). Today, with the increasing ease and accessibility of various forms of telecommunication, client confidentiality can be easily and unintentionally compromised, as art therapists capture and transmit artwork in digital formats (Orr 2012). Further, when art is produced in an art therapy session, for example, it is not always clear how therapists should respond when clients want to give the artwork away.

Other ethical dilemmas can arise with the complexity of art content. Art therapists encourage clients to express themselves in deeply personal ways and the unfiltered subject matter that manifests in client artwork can present unique challenges that do not appear in other forms of psychotherapy. Provocative themes of aggression, sexuality, and spirituality can emerge silently in artwork without awareness by the client; still, the content must be addressed in treatment, sometimes by direct interpretation and other times by unspoken acknowledgement. Art therapists must make these responses without imparting personal bias or self-motivated interventions. Provocative imagery in art can be as clinically significant as overt behavior in a session, yet there is little guidance in professional standards or in educational settings on how this content should be addressed.

Other awkward dilemmas in the ethical practice of art therapy can occur with the use of art materials as an integral part of treatment. Working with art supplies sometimes places art therapists in close physical proximity or contact with clients which does not occur in more traditional forms of therapy, and it can be easily misconstrued. With all of these unique considerations in the practice of art therapy, there are few specific guidelines for physical contact, giving or receiving artwork as gifts, or the digital transmission of artwork, and sometimes what is written is vague or conflicted. Nonetheless, familiarizing oneself with federal, state, institutional, and professional ethical guidelines is the first step to clarity. There are ways to manage challenging situations in an art therapy session, with some responses more suitable than others from both a clinical and ethical perspective. When guidelines are vague or imprecise, the therapist's internal belief system can help navigate through an ethical professional quandary (Kapitan 2011; Moon 2006; Trevino and Brown 2004).

One of the best ways to build a strong sense of internal ethics is to pay attention when unusual physical feelings arise around ethical dilemmas. Feeling anxious, ashamed, uncomfortable, or reluctant to share your decision or situation with others may indicate a conflict with one's sense of values or principles. Identifying these feelings is the first step to awareness and consistency of ethical action. When a confusing situation presents itself, a therapist must find a trusted mentor, peer, or colleague to discuss the issue further, without fear, shame, or professional retribution, allowing for a positive rather than fear-driven learning experience with ethical dilemmas (Hinz 2011). Positive mentorship, especially in a supervisory relationship is crucial to fostering ethical conduct. Studies have shown that supervisors with strong, well-developed standards of conduct can greatly influence supervisees, making them less likely to engage in unethical behavior (Pope, Tabachnik, and Keith-Spiegel 1987; Trevino and Brown 2004). Along the path of experience, most, if not all, therapists will make choices that, while driven by the best of intentions, are less than perfect. Yet, with insight and motivation for change, a questionable choice has the power to be transformed into a valuable learning experience, even if the lesson is to not make that particular choice again.

## Mandatory vs. aspirational ethics

Ethics are an integral part of the helping profession because of the inherent sense of responsibility that comes with effecting actions on others. All standards of helping professions practices embrace the understanding that clinicians do no harm to clients. Without guilt, concern, or fear of the potential harm to others there would be no ethical dilemmas or sense of accountability (Newman, Gray, and Fuqua 1996). In an attempt to minimize these conflicts, most standards of practice develop guidelines that reflect *mandatory* ethics. Mandatory ethics dictate a minimal standard, generally reflecting legal guidelines, by which one must practice, i.e., not having sexual relationships with or engaging in exploitive relationships with clients. These kinds of guidelines provide a measure by which to assess, enforce, and standardize behaviors specific to a given profession, but they can be limiting as they do not encourage higher levels of accountability and competence (Newman *et al.* 1996).

*Aspirational* ethics, on the other hand, are the utmost standards to which a professional practice can attain (Corey, Schneider-Corey, and Callanan 2007). A practitioner's aspirational ethics go beyond what is simply legally compliant to encompass all aspects of practice which affect the well being of the client. Seeking an aspirational approach to ethics suggests motivation and intent beyond the minimal requirements, thereby promoting a higher level of professional practice (Newman *et al.*1996). For art therapists, this higher level of professional standard can be cultivated by continued engagement in post-graduate educational experiences, examining personal issues that may impact professional practice and embracing leadership and art therapy advocacy roles in legislature and the community at large (Hinz 2011).

The concept of aspirational ethics is particularly important to art therapists because the practice is so complex. The fusion of art, symbolism, and expression in a form of psychotherapy will always require a deeper, more elaborate exploration of ethical practice because of the complex and subjective nature of the artistic content and the physically interactive nature of the art process. Standards of practice alone will never address each and every ethical issue, so art therapists must develop an internalized, evolved standard of professionalism based on personal integrity and virtue (Hinz 2011; Kapitan 2011).

## Beneficence and competence

Most therapists are truly motivated by an honorable internal desire to do what is right and good. This altruism, or *beneficence*, is often driven by a high degree of personal insight and an aptitutde for self-discerning objectivity which is enhanced by maturity and professional experience. Selflessness, with a focus on the needs of the client, demands consideration for all of the diverse aspects of the personal, cultural, and ethnic qualities that define individuals. Beneficence also evolves from an empathic awareness of the needs of the individual and the community, which ultimately inspires more permanent societal change (Meara, Schmidt, and Day 1996). Being faithful, loyal, and truthful are characteristics of strong moral character as well as important traits for ethical professional practice. Developing these traits makes it easier to make sound professional choices when presented with ethical challenges (Koocher and Keith-Spiegel 2008).

In addition to an aspiration towards beneficence, most ethical guidelines also stipulate that therapists only practice within their professional scope of clinical competence. Not surprisingly, there is a mutually dependent relationship between beneficence and competence. If therapists practice outside of their level of knowledge or ability, whether intentional or not, it is likely that harm will be done. Moreover, professional competence is difficult to measure. There are several aspects to consider, including educational, clinical, intellectual, and emotional competence (Welfel 2006). Clinical competence embodies educational knowledge in the field of practice, plus a refined level of expertise and diligence to maintain that expertise. Intellectual and educational competence implies a level of education in specialized areas within a specific discipline, as well as the strategies to apply that knowledge (Welfel 2006).

Knowledge and skill capacity are only a part of competency in practice. Emotional competence is also important in ethical practice, combining an ability to understand and express feelings that are both objective and situationally appropriate in the therapeutic setting, while managing any personal prejudice (Pope, Sonne, and Greene 2006). An ability to express traits such as self-control and self-confidence contributes to a higher level of emotional competence and ultimately an increased ability to relate to clients (Kak, Berkhalter, and Cooper 2001). For art therapists, the art process itself can inform this level of emotional awareness, or ethos, as it can bypass defenses and allow for a greater awareness in understanding clients and their conflicts (Kapitan 2011).

Professional competence in art therapy may also include experience working with particular art materials, such as welding or kiln-fired pottery, which require specific knowledge to ensure safety as well as the capacity to impart this complex skill to clients. Specialized areas of expertise in art therapy can also include experience with a population with specific needs, such as the deaf and blind or individuals with complex medical challenges. Unfortunately, requirements for deeming one experienced in a specialty area vary greatly, calling for greater continuity and specificity within credentialing authorities in this area (Packard, Simon, and Vaughn 2006). Nonetheless, it is the responsibility of the art therapist to be diligent in acquiring the necessary proficiency and experience before practicing in a special area. Practitioners should be honest, using full transparency to inform clients of their level of experience in a specific area *before* treatment.

## Competence and credentials

Informing clients of education and training can lower liability risks. Practicing outside the scope of practice can make art therapists vulnerable to accusations of breach of contract or malpractice, as well as complaints of insufficient training (Kak, Berkhalter, and Cooper 2001). Aside from possible legal implications if a formal complaint is filed, there is an implied ethical responsibility on the part of therapists to achieve and maintain proficiency in an area of practice. Additionally, making information available about training and areas of expertise allows clients to make informed choices (ATCB 2011, § 3.5.1). Both the Art Therapy Credentials Board (ATCB) (2011 § 3.5.2), and the American Art Therapy Association (AATA) (2011 § 5.0–5.7 and §11.6) require art therapists to accurately represent their credentials, educational training, and areas of expertise. AATA's ethical principles go on to say that accurate representation extends to any promotional materials or advertisements (AATA 2011, § 11.3).

AATA ethical guidelines are also currently under revision to clarify more specifically how unregistered, unlicensed and/

or non-certified graduates from an accredited program should represent themselves. Should they be called art therapists and promote themselves as such? Is simply graduating from an accredited program sufficient training to practice with competence in the field? Art therapist registered (ATR) and board certification (BC) are voluntary credentials awarded by the national organizing body of the ATCB. The ATCB has a mission of maintaining, overseeing, and monitoring the credentials and standards of professional competence for art therapists. The AATA provides education and awareness of the standards of practice for art therapy. Both organizations work hand in hand to differentiate the practice of art therapy from other therapy or counseling professions, as a mental health profession which utilizes the application of established principles of human development, social development, counseling theory, and art techniques (AATA 2011; ATCB 2011). Therefore, obtaining registration and certification support a higher standard of ethical and professional practice.

Graduation from an accredited program is the first step towards achieving professional competency but it does not necessarily mean graduates are ready to practice competently without guidance (Kitzrow 2002). In order to maintain a high standard of professional competence, art therapy registration requires graduates to obtain a certain amount of direct client contact while supervised by an art therapist in order to accumulate professional experience before practicing independently. Board certification requires testing in addition, raising the standards further. It is possible to practice in some states without registration, if a therapist is working in an institutional setting under supervision with a licensed clinician or with a limited permit that implies an ultimate goal of licensure. Some states require licensing in order to practice psychotherapy. These state laws supersede any less stringent national guidelines, and licensing is mandatory for clinical practice of any kind in those states.

Some art therapists feel graduating from an accredited program is sufficient and do not pursue further credentials. They may attempt to practice without registration or licensing in states where the credentialing standards are vague, but this behavior does not support maintaining high standards of ethical art therapy practice. Additionally, obtaining proper credentials is an important way to quickly know a therapist's educational training, especially on abbreviated promotional materials, such as business cards and pamphlets. When credential letters appear after an art therapist's name, one can be sure he has graduated from an accredited art therapy program. Just listing a graduating degree or certificate does not imply that the program is accredited by AATA, nor is it realistic for a consumer to know which programs are accredited art therapy programs. Credentials easily verify that an art therapist has graduated from an accredited program with all of the necessary educational training.

In summary, if art therapists want the same clinical status as other mental health practitioners, we must, as a profession, maintain standards of practice by applying for any and all appropriate post-graduate credentials. The AATA (2012) position statement regarding licensure for art therapists supports any regulations and policies on the federal and state level that encourage efforts to obtain licensing of art therapists. Support of AATA's position should begin with *all* practicing art therapists becoming registered, board certified, and licensed, where applicable, to ensure professional competency and the highest standards of professional practice.

## Challenges in the ethical decision making process

Challenges in the ethical practice of art therapy generally arise when awkward topics are not clearly defined in institutional and organizational guidelines, or when there is a conflict between these guidelines and personal value systems. Sometimes an ethical challenge arises due to a conflict between the therapist's personal needs and the therapeutic goals for a client. This is the time when supervision, peer support, or collegial guidance is most helpful, but it may not be available in the moment when ethical decisions must be made. While these conflictual situations are infrequent, and the motivations are well intended, the practitioner's choices may be lacking in guidance and clarity.

Other times, ethical conflicts arise consistently with the same individuals. With students, repeated ethical quandaries may be related to a lack of experience or maturity as a clinician and they generally respond well to mentorship and guidance. Seasoned therapists, however, who repeatedly exhibit unethical or unprincipled professional behavior suggest something different. These individuals generally exhibit characteristics such as a general ignorance of professional ethical standards and poor personal or professional boundaries. They may seem preoccupied, unaware, inattentive, or irresponsible, displaying a lack of empathy for their clients and a general inability to put their clients' needs and therapeutic goals before their own (Koocher and Keith-Spiegel 2008). Often these clinicians do not actively seek out peer support or mentorship on their own.

Aside from a lack of awareness, fears about the repercussions over breaches of ethics can create distrustful environments, promoting shame or fear and discouraging practitioners from seeking ethical guidance. Ironically, this response seems at odds with what sound ethical practice attempts to promote: confidence, empowerment, and trust. Recently, a more positive approach has evolved when addressing breaches of ethics. Many supervisors and experienced practitioners have begun to embrace an affirmative approach to ethical practice with the hope of encouraging a practitioner to seek guidance as well as an impetus for learning and behavior change (Hinz 2011).

Another current model for addressing growth in ethical practice focuses on ways to identify an individual's willingness to change persistent, less effective ways of practice (Kak, Berkhalter and Cooper 2001; Prochaska, Norcross, and

DiClemente 1995). The stages of readiness for change include pre-stages of contemplation and preparation which are marked by attempts to increase knowledge. In this way, mentorship and educational awareness, along with motivation, can change persistent negative and unethical practice. A willingness to change is crucial in the process of strengthening healthier and more productive behaviors. In the context of ethics, a readiness for change model can help practitioners prepare for higher aspirations of ethical practice in the face of unclear situations.

Willingness to change is generally ingrained in the art therapy student's commitment to complete his degree requirements and can be easily integrated into the graduate level curriculum as part of the internship and supervisory process. Motivation to continue to learn and maintain skill levels is more challenging with experienced practitioners and should be encouraged with peer support and advocacy. For supervisors and art therapy educators, ways to increase competency and ethical practice in art therapy can include encouraging participation in continuing education courses, lectures, and conferences, which are optimal ways to stay up to date on the latest trends in practice. In addition, accessibility of online learning tools and internet-based courses makes self-education a popular method of continued learning and increased professional competence (Kak, Berkhalter and Cooper 2001). Most importantly, mentoring and the trusted supervisory relationship that includes case reviews and in-depth monitoring of therapist-client relationships can provide the most powerful incidental learning experiences through modeling and trust-based incidental learning (Trevino and Brown 2004).

Ethical practice in art therapy includes an awareness of how the delicate balance between competence, the artistic process, the therapeutic relationship, and the art space combine to create an ideal healing experience for clients (Moon 2006). Experience and empathy allow the art therapist to know when to focus on a discussion of the art, when to simply allow the art process to take over, and when to utilize the benefits of a safe space to create (Moon 2006). Peer support, mentorship, and continued willingness to change and grow as a practitioner will maintain high standards of ethical practice in the face of challenging ethical situations.

## When confronted with an ethical challenge...

- Pay attention to uncomfortable feelings you may be experiencing.

- Familiarize yourself with federal, state, and professional guidelines.

- Determine if there is a conflict between personal values and the professional guidelines.

- Determine if the dilemma has legal as well as ethical consequences.

- Identify all individuals who would be affected by your decision.

- Identify all possible outcomes.

- Assess the level of benefit or harm that may occur.

- Seek guidance from a trusted supervisor, mentor, or colleague.

CHAPTER I

# Sexuality in the Therapeutic Environment

## Introduction

The topic of sexuality, by its very nature, is awkward and made even more so when viewed in the context of the therapeutic relationship. Sexuality manifested in any therapy setting is a theme largely absent from the curriculum of clinical training programs and the subject is only scantly addressed in literature (Pope *et al.* 2006; Pope, Tabachnick, and Keith-Spiegel 1986). In addition, sexuality is not often considered within the context of cultural norms of both the therapist and the client (Talwar 2010). What may be sexually acceptable in one culture may be deeply insulting or embarrassing in another. Art therapists, in particular, may have a more complicated experience addressing sexuality in therapy. Not only can sexuality be expressed verbally or behaviorally in the art therapy session, but also more directly in the art content. Depending on the therapist's response to sexual art content, sexual expression in client art can further complicate therapeutic goals and the client-therapist relationship.

With so much to consider, there is no one correct answer or approach when addressing sexual topics in therapy. Rather, there are a number of variables to consider within the ethical and legal principles of the art therapy profession and the stylistic approach of the therapist. Awkward as it may be, here one finds a challenging dilemma with only one place to start: art therapists must first and foremost honestly explore their own feelings about sexuality. Specifically, they should consider how they are most comfortable expressing these feelings themselves. For example, what are their personal feelings about sexuality and sexual orientation? Do these feelings reflect social norms? Are they more physically or verbally expressive in their sexuality? When they feel sexually attracted to someone, do they touch them more? Do they speak to them in a different way? Do they dress differently? Noticing these preferences can help identify when an art therapist may be experiencing or responding to sexuality in a therapeutic context with clients.

It is also important to remember that humans are sexual beings by nature. Procreation is the survival mechanism of our species and humans attach complex feelings to the sexual act, shaped by social and cultural influences (Jackson and Scott 2010; Masters and Johnson 1981). Exploring sexual preference, gender, and sexual expression are a normal part of human development which generally begins in adolescence and continues throughout adulthood (Blos 1979). Discovering one's sexuality is a personal experience that will enhance professional growth as an empathic clinician. Therapists comfortable exploring their own sexual orientation or sexual trauma may, under certain conditions, find they have particular empathy for client populations with sexual issues. However, under different circumstances, these personal experiences may limit their ability to practice with these populations. There is no clearly defined protocol for exploring one's past. The journey of discovery, however, should occur outside of the therapeutic setting, in personal therapy, clinical supervision, or under the guidance of a trusted mentor but never in the context of the therapeutic relationship with clients.

Art therapists must also consider these expressions within the guidelines of ethical behavior. Sexual harassment, sexual contact, or any other kind of sexually exploitive behaviors are never permitted, as outlined in the art therapy and other professional discipline code of ethics for obvious reasons of potential client harm (Behnke 2006), but more subtle sexual expression and how it manifests in the therapeutic relationship is not as clearly defined. Most frequently, art therapy students and new graduates will ask about whether or not to hug a client, how to deflect flirtatious client behavior, or how to respond to sexually explicit artwork made in sessions. Less often, and usually with encouragement, students and practicioners may ask about how to deal with sexual feelings towards clients. All of these topics are a normal part in the development of a therapeutic relationship, especially with client populations that struggle with sexual issues. It is imperative to have supportive, professional supervision or mentorship to discuss these complicated issues. Given thoughtful attention to all of these considerations and a supportive supervisory setting, with time and experience art therapists will develop stylistically comfortable ways to acknowledge, redirect, process, and explore sexual behavior and art content in the therapeutic setting.

## Sexual feelings toward clients

One survey of 575 psychotherapists revealed that 95 percent of male and 76 percent of female therapists admitted to, at least once, having sexual feelings for their clients (Pope *et al.* 1986). Sixty three percent felt guilty, anxious, or confused about the attraction. About half of the respondents did not receive any guidance or training concerning this issue, and only 9 percent reported that their training or supervision in this area was adequate.

While sexual attraction toward a client is considered a common experience that can be addressed without interfering with the therapeutic goals, more intense sexualized feelings can be harmful. A therapist's sexual preoccupation with a client can create loss of clarity and objectivity as well as distract from treatment goals. When the client becomes a sexualized object, a therapist may have difficulty experiencing empathy which can ultimately cause confusion in roles/boundaries/fantasy and reality. Oftentimes, a therapist's personal conflicts can contribute to escalating sexual feelings towards clients, making objectivity in treatment even more difficult (Ladany *et al.* 1997).

Over 500 therapists were surveyed and reported that they were most sexually attracted to clients that displayed specific traits such as physical attractiveness along with some kind of above average levels of intelligence or cognition, as well as some level of vulnerability. In addition, the therapists reported perceiving some type of sexual behavior on the part of the client (Pope, Tabachnick and Keith-Speige 1987). In a classroom or supervisory setting, it is not uncommon to hear art therapy students and supervisees report that they feel sexually attracted to clients that exhibit above average levels of artistic ability. As highly creative individuals, art therapists tend to find these same traits appealing and this may add to the romantic attraction to a client. Not surprisingly, these traits—physical attractiveness, vulnerability, intelligence, and, for art therapists, high levels of artistic creativity—could also be described as the same qualities they may seek in romantic partners.

## CASE SCENARIO

A 27-year-old art therapy intern in her second year of training in a masters level program, reported feeling confusing feelings about a male client diagnosed with post traumatic stress disorder and substance abuse issues in an outpatient treatment facility for veterans. She described this client as being generally more insightful and artistically talented than other program participants and reported that he often gave her small gifts such as shells, small stones, art postcards, and sometimes artwork he produced in session. Although the client was approximately 30 years older than herself, the therapist reported she found the client sexually attractive and that she often thought about him outside of sessions, fantasizing about him as a romantic partner and comparing him to her fiancé, whom she planned to marry later in the year. She haltingly revealed in group supervision that she found herself concocting reasons to prolong treatment sessions, although her client had met treatment goals, solely because of her sexual attraction to him.

In group supervision, the intern was first commended for her ability to acknowledge her feelings and bring the issue into the context of supervision for support and guidance, rather than allowing these feelings to further affect her objectivity. Using artwork, personal therapy, and discussion with peers, she was encouraged to explore her current relationship with her boyfriend and consider how, if at all, it may have contributed to the emergence of sexualized feelings towards her client. The following week, the intern reported that she believed anxiety about her upcoming marriage and her fiancé's ability to provide for her had contributed to her sexualized feelings towards her client. Once this connection was made, she was able to more objectively focus on termination treatment goals for her client.

## Managing sexual feelings toward clients

Sexual feelings towards clients are unavoidable. Embarrassment often keeps therapists from discussing these feelings and it is important to remember that these feelings, while normal, are not helpful in the therapeutic setting. Additionally, when therapists feel vulnerable or are struggling with personal issues, they are more likely to unknowingly manifest sexualized feelings towards clients (Amos and Margison 2006; Butler and Zelen 1977; Fisher 2004). Knowing how to recognize these common feelings, acknowledge them, and seek support demonstrates ethical responsibility and maturity in clinical practice.

**Consider the following to determine whether or not your sexual feelings towards a client may inhibit treatment goals or the development of an appropriate therapeutic relationship:**

- Are you consciously dressing in a particular way when you are scheduled to see a particular client?

- Do you have recurrent daydreams, fantasies, or sexual thoughts about a certain client?

- Are you inclined to ask a client personal questions that are not treatment goal related, hoping that you have shared interests?

- Are you flirtatious in your body language or tone of voice?

- Do you feel an urge to discuss sexually explicit material or make sexual references when it is not treatment goal related?

- Are your sexually stimulated by the content of your client's artwork? Do you view this artwork for the purposes of sexual stimulation outside of the treatment setting?

- Are you sexually aroused when you think about this client or see the client in a session?

- Are you distracted with these private thoughts while in the presence of this client?

Having sexual thoughts about clients and acting on these thoughts are very different, the former being expected and the latter causing significant harm (Fisher 2004). Research and clinical experience show that even revealing these feelings generally makes the client feel uncomfortable or can make the client think the disclosure is an invitation to relax professional boundaries or pursue a sexual relationship (Fisher 2004). It is imperative to seek outside support to manage these sexual feelings rather than burden a client with a self-disclosure.

To gain greater insight into sexual feelings and the associated discomfort and embarrassment, discuss feelings with someone with professional experience whom you trust. Additionally, supervisors and educators should create an environment that allows supervisees to comfortably discuss sexual topics without fear of appearing provocative (Pope *et al.* 2006). Supervisors should also be alert to incidental supervisee disclosure that may be attempts to discuss more significant issues around sexuality.

## CASE SCENARIO

A female graduate art therapy student in her early fifties reported in supervision that she had been struggling with an art therapy group of male veterans that lacked cohesion with members losing interest shortly after the start of the group. After exploring possible reasons for the stagnant group dynamic, including the types of art therapy directives and materials, the student described one member in the group, approximately ten years her junior, with whom she felt particularly connected. She described giving individual attention to this member in the group because she felt she had a great deal in common with this member, particularly after discovering they had attended the same high school. In addition, she reported feeling a kinship with him as he came from the same cultural and socio-economic background, finally admitting, that under different circumstances, he was the kind of man she probably would have dated in high school. With this admission, she was able to acknowledge feeling sexually attracted to this member and being pleased he responded to her attention in the group. The supervision group members helped her see that her need to connect with this member did not effectively serve the group as a whole, and additionally, the group deterioration and subsequent lack of cohesion may have been influenced by the other group members' awareness of her inability to equalize her attention towards all group members.

---

## Sexual contact between therapist and client

Thinking about clients in a sexual context and acting on these feelings are two very different situations. Statistically, self-reporting surveys suggest that as many as 12 percent of therapists have or have had sexual relationships with clients (Lamb and Catanzaro 1998; Lamb *et al.* 2003; Pope 1993). Any kind of sexual physical contact can have a devastating effect on the welfare of a client, hence the clear ethical and legal guidelines on this topic (Pope 2001). Clients come to the therapeutic relationship in a vulnerable state, seeking support, mentorship, and guidance during emotionally challenging times. Often their ability to make appropriate judgments is impaired, making them at risk of harm if they were to enter into a confusing relationship with a therapist (Pope 2001). Additionally, because of the fiduciary, or trust-based, nature of the client-therapist relationship, it would be highly unethical for a therapist to derive sexual pleasure from the client, given the potential for harm (Behnke 2006). Phyllis Chesler (2005), in her landmark book, *Women and Madness*, described some of the harmful effects of therapist and client sexual intimacy, including cognitive dysfunction, emotional lability, an impaired ability to trust, increased suicidal risk, and sexual confusion. Because this kind of relationship also violates personal and professional boundaries, clients may also experience responses similar to other forms of sexual abuse (Kluft 1989; Pope 1990; Sonne and Pope 1991).

## Client initiated sexuality

Clients who are in the midst of trauma or high levels of stress are at risk for confusing nurturing or caretaking in the therapeutic relationship for sexual or romantic interest on the part of the therapist. In particular, clients who are psychotic, delusional, developmentally delayed, addicted, victims of sexual trauma, or in early stages of grief are particularly vulnerable to expressing sexuality as a means of intensifying attachment to the therapist. While on some level this can be flattering for the therapist, it is extremely important to reinstate an appropriate client/therapist boundary by reminding the client that sexual relationships in treatment are inappropriate. As with other awkward situations with clients, rebuffing romantic overtures or addressing sexually explicit content in art is tricky. Tact, grace, and empathy will reinforce boundaries while preserving the therapeutic relationship.

---

### CASE SCENARIO

On an inpatient unit for substance abuse treatment, an experienced art therapist observed one of the male patients flirting openly and making blatant sexual comments to a young art therapy intern under her supervision. The student, visibly uncomfortable and unable to respond to the client, looked to the supervisor for support. In an attempt to model an appropriate response without shaming the client, the supervisor said, "I can see that you are very interested in our intern and what you are saying and doing is making her feel uncomfortable. I am going to remind you to stay focused on your treatment goals while in the art therapy group." If the behavior continued, the supervisor stated that she would ask the client to leave the group. Following the session, the supervisor met with the intern to discuss the issue to determine if she would be comfortable setting limits in this way should the situation arise in the future.

---

## CASE SCENARIO

A young art therapy student in her twenties interning at an inpatient psychiatric facility was walking back to the art therapy room to put away art supplies. As she passed by a patient, she noticed he had opened his pants and was exposing himself to her. Shocked, she did not acknowledge the behavior. Later, she found the same client crouched outside of her office door as she was leaving for the day. Again, she did not acknowledge the behavior. She knew that this client, diagnosed with paranoid schizophrenia, also had a history of violence towards women and lived in her neighborhood. Over the next few days, she became increasingly more anxious about her safety, avoidant of the patient, and concerned he would attend her groups and harass her. Eventually she reported the behavior to a supervisor and the clinical team, including the chief psychiatrist, psychologist, case worker, and support staff, confronted the client and directed him to cease the behavior. There were no more incidents and the art therapist felt supported by her team of colleagues.

## Sexual content in art

The following three case scenarios describe some typical ways sexual content is manifested in artwork. Sexual content in artwork can be both shocking and stimulating at the same time and how the sexual content is managed can have a powerful impact on treatment. Oftentimes, lack of experience or confidence and their own sexual values may prevent a therapist from responding at all, which can add to the confusion of the situation. While there is no one right way to always handle sexual content in art, there are some guidelines that may assist in managing responses.

## CASE SCENARIO

An art therapist in an after school program for at risk children described a group discussion about the recent and rather sudden departure of the previous art therapist. The all-male members spontaneously began to describe feelings of sadness and anger around the loss of the therapist. One nine-year-old boy in the group, however, did not know the previous therapist and appeared to feel left out of the conversation, as evidenced by his quiet demeanor and lack of verbal interaction. Suddenly, without any warning, the boy drew a large penis on the art table. Needless to say, the ongoing conversation stopped and laughter erupted.

## CASE SCENARIO

A 22-year-old male was living at home with his parents after a difficult year at college. In his first art therapy session, the client appeared agitated, distracted, and unfocused. When asked to draw anything he liked, he made a pencil drawing of six androgynous couples in various sexual positions of coitus and fellatio. Without a word, he handed the completed drawing to the art therapist.

## CASE SCENARIO

An art therapist, working with adults diagnosed with chronic schizophrenia in a community based treatment facility, noted that her clients' artwork often revealed a great deal of sexual content. Some of the content was obvious but not offensive, such as figures with exaggerated breasts and excessive detailing in the pelvic area whereas other content was more symbolically represented. For example, clients might sexualize what would otherwise be common, generally non-sexual objects such as magic wands, hotdogs, and skyscrapers. The clients seemed unaware of the sexualized content and it was rarely, if ever, addressed in art therapy groups.

In each of these three case scenarios, sexual content in the art is evident, yet the therapeutic context of the creation of the images is quite different, as are the treatment goals and developmental stage of each client, both of which must be considered before making any kind of intervention. In the first case, the nine-year-old boy seemed to create the image as a means of diverting attention from the difficult topic of loss and anger around the loss of the group's previous therapist. He may have felt left out of the conversation because he never knew the therapist or, as a new member in the program, he may have felt uncomfortable with the deep level of emotional content of the discussion. In either case, an appropriate intervention would focus on the content of the art as disruptive to the group discussion and whether or not this was an appropriate way to seek attention. Feeling alienated, feeling uncomfortable expressing difficult feelings appropriately, and seeking alternatives to negative attention seeking behaviors are all common therapeutic goals when working with conduct disordered children and this would have been an appropriate treatment goal with this child. Once this brief intervention was made, the conversation could return to the feelings about the departed therapist with all members engaged.

In the second example, the 22-year-old male was straddling two important developmental stages that explore the formation of one's own identity and seeking intimacy in relationships (Erikson 1993). Since developmental stages are fluid, it is possible that this young man was also still exploring aspects of the previous stages of adolescent identity development, an aspect of which often includes exploration of sexual identity both in terms of gender preference as well as the relationship between sexuality and intimacy (Blos 1979; Erikson 1993).

With this in mind, it seemed important to reflect back to the client the impact of his drawing on the therapist's first impression of him. Remarking that the drawing's subject was highly intimate yet depersonalized by the cartoonish representation, it might seem that he was making a strong statement about intimacy and one way to shield against possible rejection, which was to remain anonymous in the sexual act. The therapist also remarked that beginning a therapeutic relationship, while it does not involve sexual intimacy, does involve a different kind of intimacy, but one that can nonetheless give rise to fears of rejection. Accepting this client's drawing as an expression of a fear of rejection, rather than focusing on the sexual content, both clarified the boundaries of the therapeutic relationship and reassured the client of his acceptance by the therapist. In this case, it was important to consider not only the stage of development of the client but also the stage of the therapeutic relationship.

The last case scenario attempted to illustrate that sexual content in the art of some psychiatric populations may be a normal expression of unfulfilled adult sexual needs. Many psychiatrically impaired adults have been mentally ill for most of their lives, with recurrent and frequent hospitalizations per year. Often unable to hold down a job or maintain friendships, their lives have remained a desolate and isolated existence, hampered by constant battles with delusional thinking and periods of psychosis. Since normal social interactions are difficult, it stands to reason that sexual intimacy is also out of reach for much of this population. Moreover, as the art therapist reported that most of her clients were highly adverse to any kind of physical touch, even non-sexual physical intimacy was problematic as well. Sometimes, the art therapist reported that the sexual content, based on a client's history, seemed related to an earlier sexual trauma and in these cases, she addressed the content in an individual session or outside of the group setting. Still, most often, it seemed that much of the sexualized content in this population's artwork was an expected and normal expression of longing for sexual intimacy. In this case, discussing the content in an art therapy group would only evoke unnecessary humiliation and shame.

## Managing sexual feelings toward clients in treatment

Sexuality in the form of expressed art content, sexual behavior by clients, and sexual feelings towards clients appear to be a common and expected occurrence, given the nature of pathology and the intensity of the client/therapist relationship, especially when working with clients that have experienced sexual trauma. Acting on sexual feelings towards clients is never acceptable, nor does admitting these feelings to a client serve any therapeutic value (Fisher 2004 ; Lamb and Catanzaro 1998; Pope 2001). Students and therapists must be open to exploring their own feelings about sexuality and touch as well as awareness of vulnerabilities in this area. Clinicians seem particularly vulnerable during times of personal romantic calamity. Sexual attraction towards clients should be metered with constraint and consultation, supervision, or support from trusted supervisors and colleagues (Ladany *et al.* 1997).

Sexual behavior and content in art can be stimulating to the therapist as the viewer. While addressing the therapist's stimulation seems to have no therapeutic value, the art content and behavior expressed by clients should be addressed in the context of treatment goals. Clients who have experienced sexual trauma or exploitation are particularly vulnerable when engaged in treatment and are most likely to express sexuality in the treatment context. Similarly, clients in normal periods of development, such as adolescence, are likely to express sexuality. Rigorous assessment can determine whether these expressions are normal or pathological in content, which will determine the type of intervention. Addressing sexual content in treatment is different from expressing a voyeuristic interest in clients' sexual activities, and therapists should genuinely examine personal and professional motivations when exploring the topic.

### In summary, avoiding these situations can assist in managing sexuality in the therapeutic setting:

- Sexual feelings towards clients are normal and expected. Sexually intimate relationships with clients, students, and supervisees are never ethically appropriate and may constitute legal violations.

- Client initiated sexuality does not excuse a therapist from maintaining professional boundaries. Practice restraint and always address these behaviors or art content in the context of therapeutic goals.

- Discussing sexual content in art or touching a client for erotic fulfillment is never justified and is highly unethical.

Because the art process provides easy access to unconscious material, art therapists will often be exposed to sexualized content in art and in the behavior of their clients. When assessing how to, if at all, acknowledge sexuality in the therapeutic environment, consider first the developmental sexual norms for the client. Assess the needs of the client population. Particularly isolated and disturbed populations, adolescents, and geriatrics will naturally express sexual content in art as it is lacking in their daily lives. When the expressed behavior or content seems dysfunctional or pathological, reiterate boundaries and seek support. Remember that sexual expression, in its healthy form, is a normal part of human behavior.

CHAPTER 2

# Ethical Considerations with Cognitively Impaired Clients

## Introduction

Clinicians must take into account a number of ethical considerations when engaging in treatment or research with cognitively impaired clients. Issues of competency, capacity, and informed consent often create ethical conundrums that are at cross purposes with therapeutic goals and client confidentiality (Appelbaum and Grisso 1988; Beattie 2007; Deaver 2011; Karlawish 2003; Kim 2011; Kim *et al.* 2005; Kim *et al.* 2009). For example, when should a clinician reveal that cognitively impaired clients are unable to care for themselves or make independent decisions? If they are unable to do so, who should make those decisions for them? If a clinician fails to report concerns about competency or capacity, is he liable for any harm that might come to the client? If a clinician reports these concerns, is he breaching client confidentiality? Mandated reporting laws more clearly articulate the legal, and to some extent, ethical guidelines regarding when a clinician should report suspected abuse or impending harm, as well as the legal consequences of not reporting (US Department of Health and Human Services 2012), but ethical practice for competency assessment and intervention is not as clearly defined.

Art therapists have additional considerations with this population because cognitive impairments and decline are often evidenced in artwork before the effects are manifested in observed behaviors (Stallings 2010; Stewart 2004); however, using artwork as a measure of predictive behavior can be risky without other supporting evidence. Still, diagnostic information from artwork, specifically in the early stages of cognitive decline, can help identify areas of need for clients and avoid potentially dangerous situations before they might occur. Artwork and the creative art process may therefore be particularly useful in assessing levels of competence and capacity.

The following case is a fascinating example of the unique and unpredictable manifestation of cognitive decline in the artwork of a well-trained artist with an unusual form of dementia. The case illuminates some of the complicated ethical considerations with cognitively impaired populations, in that inconsistent levels of declining cognition make assessment of capacity sometimes confounding. Because of the high level of involvement of the subject's husband, the case also highlights the value of having an involved caregiver as a surrogate in the decision making process. Most importantly, the therapist may come to understand that when a client's cognitive impairment affects the expressive language centers, it does not necessarily reflect a client's lack of receptive language, awareness, or decision making capacities, nor their ability to engage in creative artistic expression. Knowing when to intervene and when to allow impaired clients to make decisions can assist in challenging ethical dilemmas as well as increase quality of life for these clients.

## CASE SCENARIO

Audrey (pseudonym), a 74-year-old Caucasian woman diagnosed with frontotemporal dementia (FTD) was a trained artist, writer, and educator with a long career as an exhibiting painter. Audrey began her artistic career in college as a printmaker but later revealed a real proficiency and passion for painting. She taught art at a state university for many years and wrote two books about the creative process which came out of her gratifying experiences as a fine arts instructor. Throughout most of her career, the content of her paintings mostly fell into the categories of ships, planes, trains machines, buildings, and scrap metal (Figure 2.1). As a prolific and successful artist, she had a multitude of art shows throughout the United States, and her work became part of permanent collections at national galleries, public libraries, and museums in the United States and Europe. Her main studio was in central Connecticut, but during the summer she worked in southern Vermont in a studio near her family's old farmhouse.

About ten years prior to her dementia diagnosis, Audrey wrote of her work:

> My paintings comment on the melancholy beauty found in relics of our industrial past. Both the literal and evocative meanings of these subjects strike a responsive chord in me and provide variations on a theme that has been central to my paintings for a long time. The relics remind us that, in our rapidly changing world, the triumphs of technology are just a moment away from obsolescence. Yet these remains of collapsed power have a strength, grace and sadness that is both eloquent and impenetrable. Transfigured by time and light, which render the ordinary extraordinary, they form a visual requiem for the industrial age. While my paintings are representational, their formal relationships are of equal concern to me. The ways in which the solids and spaces interact, the visual complexities of the shadows, and the changing surface qualities are all important considerations in each composition.

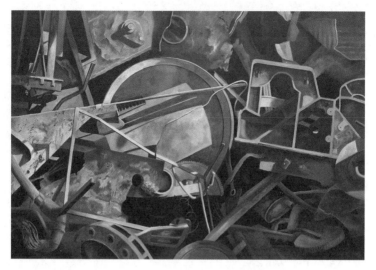

*Figure 2.1 Scrap metal, oil on canvas, 43" × 62"*
*Source: Audrey (1990)*

Several years prior to her diagnosis, Audrey's husband, Gary, began to notice concerning symptoms. About this time period, he stated:

> Because [Audrey's] mother had had Alzheimer's the possibility that [Audrey] might get it, too, lurked in the background for many years… I began to pick up expressions and gestures that reminded me of her mother's when the disease began to manifest itself in her. I was apprehensive and began a clandestine conversation with [Audrey's] doctor. After several months of denial and hiding my fears, her doctor and I decided to inform her with our concerns. It was a moment of release and relief for everyone, as [Audrey] told us how frightened she was too. Later that year she was diagnosed with dementia.

There are several types of dementia and accurate diagnosis in the early stages can be difficult. Alzheimer's disease, Lewy Body, and Creutzfeldt Jakob's diseases, often have a late age of onset, usually after the age of 60 years, and memory impairments emerge as the primary initial symptom. Fontotemporal dementia, however, affects the frontal and anterior temporal lobes, initially affecting decision making, emotional regulation, and language rather than the memory processes, thus often making it challenging to diagnose. Early symptoms may include decreased verbal expression, mood lability, personality changes, and compulsive or perseverative behaviors. Specifically, some patients may exhibit symptoms of depression, anxiety, and bizarre somatic preoccupations. Patients may also gradually become more remote, indifferent, and seemingly apathetic about people and circumstances that previously held meaning for them (Rascovsky et al. 2005; Rascovsky et al. 2011; Vandenberghe 2011).

Around the time Audrey's husband first noticed some of the early symptoms of FTD, Audrey, once a prolific painter, also began to lose interest in making art. When she did paint, according to her husband, her work demonstrated poorly organized compositions, a decreased ability to represent spatial relationships, and a lack of confidence in her brushstrokes. He also stated that she became "...convinced that her painting style was loosening and starting to look 'sloppy'" and yet, there was also a certain freedom of expression that was not present in the somewhat more rigid analytical style of the earlier works (Figure 2.2).

Similar to the relaxing of her painting style, Gary also noted at this time a shift in Audrey's behaviors. She seemed freer to express affection and less inhibited in conversations, often blurting out thoughts and comments, traits he felt were very unlike her. He noticed other changes as well, such as she began missing appointments, needing explanations for why something needed to be done, and a general lack of interest in activities that she once enjoyed. While Audrey still continued to read a great deal, she became less able to describe the content of what she was reading. More concerning, Gary also noticed an increase in paranoid thinking, as Audrey now expressed fears of intruders and began to perseverate on thoughts about setting the security alarm, locking doors, and repeatedly checking the security of their home. Audrey also began to have difficulty sleeping and became hesitant in making decisions.

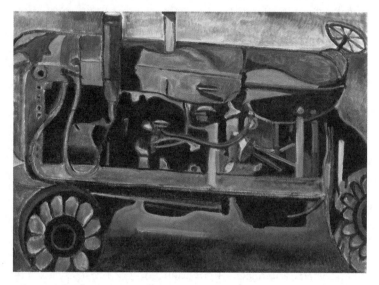

*Figure 2.2 Blue tractor, oil on canvas, 25" × 18"*
*Source: Audrey (March 2011)*

In an attempt to encourage Audrey to renew her interest in art, Gary asked a friend and artist to come to the home several times a week to assist Audrey in drawing and painting, offering her still life and photo references to work from. Audrey quickly engaged in the process and began creating several new works of art a week, though they were quite different from her earlier work. With flattened perspective, a lack of integration, and condensation of imagery, Audrey's art looked similar to the work of a child 10 to 12 years of age (Figure 2.3), depicting a limited awareness of perspective and spatial relationships as well as a limited ability to integrate objects into the surrounding environment (Lowenfeld and Brittain 1987; Malchiodi 1998). Compared to Audrey's earlier art, the work regressed in development, as evidenced by less sophisticated line quality, a limited use of color, and a more simplistic composition, typical of individuals in the moderate stage of dementia and FTD (Crutch, Isaacs, and Rossor 2001; Miller and Hou 2004; Stewart 2004).

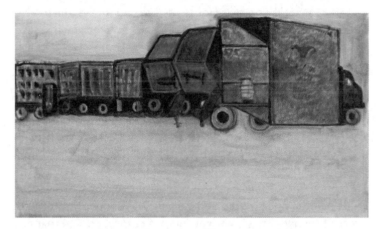

*Figure 2.3 Trucks parked in a row, oil on canvas, 28" × 16"*
*Source: Audrey (April 2011)*

Around this time, Audrey was officially diagnosed with FTD. Though always suspected, when finally confirmed by doctors, Audrey's diagnosis came as both a relief and devastation. While Gary was relieved that her symptoms were acknowledged, the prognosis for an FTD patient was grim. Typically, FTD patients submit to a rapid deterioration in cognitive functioning, including radical changes in expressive functioning. While visuospatial skills are minimally affected until later in the illness, eventually they deteriorate, along with physical functions including loss of control over bowel and bladder. Other organ functions deteriorate and immobility sets in. Death often follows as a result of pneumonia or other complications from immobility.

Generally, the progression of FTD is quicker than other forms of dementia (Rascovsky *et al.* 2005; Roberson *et al.* 2005).

Audrey's deterioration was rapid and true to the prescribed course of the illness. Approximately three years after first noticing symptoms, Audrey's husband observed dramatic changes in his wife's behavior. Most notably, she had virtually lost her capacity for expressive language, becoming as he described, "largely silent," rarely speaking or making any kind of vocalization. Still, she occasionally answered in the affirmative to express a preference. In addition, he noticed an increase in perseverative behaviors such as pacing. Audrey would track around the perimeter of their large kitchen, making right angle turns at each corner with military precision, stopping only when her attention was diverted.

Her artwork at this time also appeared different, showing a perseveration of line, pattern, and schema (Figure 2.4). She would often repeatedly outline a form, much like her repetitious pacing, ceasing again only when the behavior was diverted. Dark, horizontal lines dominated the compositions of her work. Her color palette, once muted and organic was suddenly saturated, almost psychedelic, with bright, intense color, a change that has been documented in the art of other FTD patients (Budrys *et al.* 2007; Drago *et al.* 2006; Miller *et al.* 1996; Miller and Hou 2004). Audrey's images appeared more bizarre in content and lacking in perspective, almost completely flat, with foreground and background compressed. Images often merged into one another, creating a condensation of form, also a feature found in the art of other FTD patients (Rankin *et al.* 2007). Over the next few months, Audrey began painting more from her imagination, abandoning her photo references, and the work took on a freedom of expression not previously observed in her earlier works.

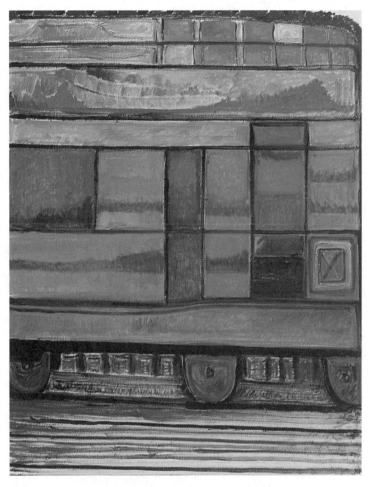

*Figure 2.4 Orange railroad car, oil on canvas, 30" × 24"*
*Source: Audrey (November 2011)*

About six months later, Audrey's husband reported that she had become fully incontinent and needed increased assistance in daily living. Her artwork production at this time was rather prolific. With encouragement, she produced at least one, and often several, drawings a day. The content of the work was bizarre and disorganized, with multiple unrelated, disconnected, and fragmented images. Often, she drew images of a horse and rider, executed in a primitive and unrefined style in pencil (Figure 2.5). The horses were often urinating or defecating, and featured enlarged or exaggerated genitalia. The inclusion of humans and animals in Audrey's work was a dramatic departure from her pre-dementia art of industrial ruins, and interestingly, all of the figures in this new work showed little or no affect. The figure's facial expression in the artwork mirrored Audrey's own blunted emotional state, suggesting a self-expressive aspect to the figures. In addition, the images seemed to lack a level of sophistication and artistic creativity that was so prevalent in her earlier works, a feature often noted in the artwork of individuals in the later stages of dementia (Flaherty 2005; Cruz de Sousa *et al.* 2010; Finney and Heilman 2007).

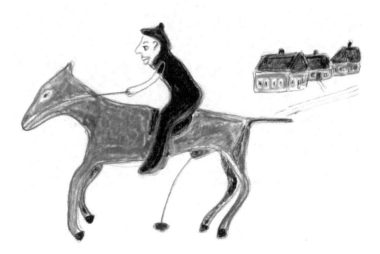

*Figure 2.5 Blue horse and rider, colored pencil on paper, 14" × 20"*
*Source: Audrey (March 2011)*

Neurologists studying FTD have observed some interesting and varied effects on creativity in individuals with previous artistic training (Budrys *et al.* 2007; Gordon 2005; Mendez 2004; Mell,

Howard, and Miller 2003; Miller *et al.* 1998; Miller and Hou 2004). Most notably, as in the case of Audrey, as expressive language and executive functions deteriorate, artists sometimes exhibit a more liberated, uninhibited style. Some neurologists believe there is a link between the expressive and receptive language areas of the brain and artistic expression, both of which are affected in FTD (Flaherty 2005; Miller and Hou 2004), and this deterioration of language functions may allow for less censorship in other areas of expression, such as in the creation of art.

Another interesting effect on creative expression in FTD patients is noted in their unusual depictions of portraits, human figures, and caricatures (Budrys *et al.* 2007; Mendez 2004). In the later stage of the illness, as patients become more dependent on caretakers, their images of humans sometimes express exaggerated, emotional expressions with themes of aggression and anxiety, almost in response to the frustration of their own lack of ability for independent functioning. At the same time, there seems to be a primitive, robotic, or mechanical quality to the expression that lacks true human expression (Budrys *et al.* 2007; Mendez 2004; Mendez and Perryman 2003; Rankin *et al.* 2007), a feature which also became more prevalent in Audrey's art.

With increased loss of control of physical functions, Audrey became more dependent on others. Her husband hired a home health aide to help care for Audrey during the day and offer some relief for himself as the sole caregiver. Audrey's artwork continued to be comprised of bizarre and intriguing images from her mind that seemed to be non-verbal expressions of her increasingly dependent state. During this time, Audrey created what Gary described as the "angry baby" picture (Figure 2.6). The figure was small in stature, wearing what appears to be a top with a bib or smock, similar to something worn by an infant or young child. The facial expression of the figure was constricted in what seemed to be frustration or anger, with arms rigid in apparent rage. It is not difficult to imagine that Audrey was poignantly expressing her frustration at her lack of self-sufficiency. The almost menacing expression on the figure's face was an expressive feature that has also been noted in the artwork of other FTD patients, along with a decrease in realism and an increase in subjective, emotional expression (Mendez 2004; Rankin *et al.* 2007).

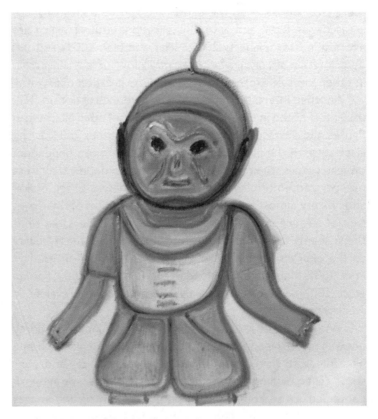

*Figure 2.6 Angry child with bib, oil on canvas, 20" × 18"*
*Source: Audrey (May 2012)*

One of the most poignant pieces Audrey created during this period seemed to movingly express the complexity of her dependent relationship with her husband (Figure 2.7). Two figures, one larger and seemingly more masculine and another more slight of frame, stand facing each other in a close embrace, looking into each other's eyes. One cannot help but surmise this entwined couple represents Audrey and her husband. What makes this piece all the more intriguing is that Gary describes Audrey, prior to her diagnosis, as not someone who was terribly passionate or sentimental, rather as someone who always exhibited a good deal of restraint. Yet, since her diagnosis, one positive outcome was Audrey's increased ability—or perhaps a disinhibition—to both accept and receive physical affection. Just as he describes in real life, in this painting there seems to be a deep emotional bond expressed in the physical connection between the two figures. Joining them at the mouth is what appears to be some kind of tube or breathing device that rises between them and disappears into the top of the page, locking the couple together in a symbiotic union. It is difficult to ignore that this artwork seems to non-verbally express Audrey's keen awareness of her deeply entwined and reliant relationship with her husband.

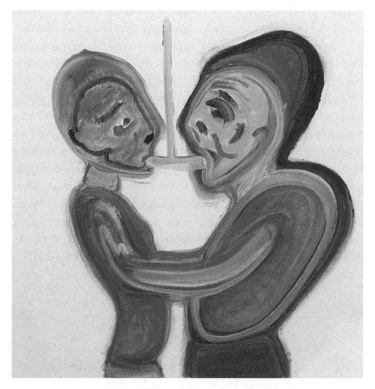

*Figure 2.7 Two figures, oil on canvas, 20" × 16"*
*Source: Audrey (May 2012)*

## COMPETENCE VS. CAPACITY

Although, in the first several years of her illness, Audrey lost a large part of her capacity for expressive language, the later art images, particularly those that display human figures, seem to suggest that she was still able to use art as a means of symbolic expression. This ability for artistic expression, along with her ability to follow directions and general compliance, suggests that while other cognitive skills diminished, her receptive language and symbolic expressive language were still intact. Her artwork also seems to suggest that she was able to understand, to some degree, her situation and surroundings, demonstrating awareness and some level of insight regarding her level of decline.

What kinds of decisions, then, should Audrey make, given her current condition? According to Gary, he and Audrey created power of attorney guidelines shortly after they were married, some 40 years prior, stipulating that either would have the ability to make business, legal, and medical decisions for each other should one of them become unable. Periodically, over the years, the parameters of the guidelines were modified to include living wills and proxy directives, reflecting ongoing support of this agreement, all of which occurred prior to Audrey's cognitive decline. Clearly in her current state, Audrey is unable to make major decisions. Yet, she still seems to have the capacity to make some daily decisions, and encouraging her to do so may help mitigate some of her evident frustration at her increasing level of dependence on others. Assessing an individual's cognitive capacity can be helpful in formulating treatment goals that can ultimately increase quality of life issues in degenerative diseases (Stewart 2004; Stallings 2010).

## Art therapy and assessing capacity

Art therapy can provide a safe forum for allowing clients independent decision making in the art process, in a way they may be unable to do so in the real world. While Audrey's case is clear in terms of her limits in functioning, other situations may be less so and warrant assessment, intervention, and support. Many types of cognitive impairment in addition to dementia, such as pervasive developmental disorders and chronic mental illness, or acute states such as active psychosis, severe anxiety, depression, mania, and late stage terminal illness, can warrant decision making surrogacy. Sometimes, medical illness can create other medical conditions such as a persistent vegetative state and coma which can also render a person's decision making skills impossible, and a proxy or surrogate should be determined. Clearly as in the case with Audrey, having a loving, invested surrogate to make medical decisions is optimal, but for most cognitively impaired clients this may not be an option.

Before clinical assessments and interventions can be made, it is important for clinicians to understand the definitions and differences of competency and capacity. A legal term, *competency*, refers to the mental ability and cognitive capabilities required to execute a legally recognized act rationally, such as standing trial, entering into a contract, or making major medical decisions, and this is determined by the court in a lengthy and complex process that takes into account a body of evidence (Buchanan 2004; Leo 1999; Resnick and Sorrentino 2005). Competency, therefore, is a global assessment of functioning.

Because there is an overlap, the term *capacity* is often confused with competency. Capacity is a functional assessment of one's ability to engage in the decision making process for a specific situation or task in the moment, and is often based on relevant demands of the environment. Simply being diagnosed with a mental illness or cognitive impairment does not automatically insinuate a lack of mental capacity (Buchanan 2004; Leo 1999). A person's capacity for decision making is based on the premise that a person understands all aspects of a given situation. For example, an individual may have the capacity to decide whether or not to have blood drawn for a test but may be incompetent to hold down a job. Global incapacity can suggest a need for a competency determination. Furthermore, capacity is not constant and it is situationally dependent, so it should be assessed over time and with a variety of measures such as the Mini Mental Status (MMSE), the MacArthur Competence Assessment Tools for Treatment (MacCAT-T) and Allen Cognitive Levels (ACLS) which use questions, interviews, and craft-based performance tasks (Allen *et al.*1992; Grisso *et al.* 1997; Reisberg *et al.* 2002).

Most cognitive assessments evaluate levels of alertness, orientation to time, place, person, and situation, all of which determine if an individual is able to engage in reality-based thinking. Levels of mental capacity will also reflect information processing, which includes immediate, short-, and long-term memory recall, all of which are needed in the course of making decisions. Sometimes, an ability to appropriately express affect can impede a person from making rational decisions or expressing preference, as may be the case in severe forms of bipolar disorder, depression, or dementia. Finally, cognitive assessments aim to determine specific areas of decline or dysfunction that may impair decision making, such as in the areas of receptive or expressive language, or planning and judgment skills (Buchanan 2004).

Clinicians must consider when an assessment is warranted. In general, clinicians agree that:

> It is not necessary to perform a formal assessment of capacity on every inpatient. For most, there is no reasonable concern for impaired capacity, obviating the need for formal testing. Likewise, in patients who clearly lack capacity, such as those with end-stage dementia or established guardians, formal reassessment usually is not required. Formal testing is most useful in situations in which capacity is unclear, disagreement

amongst surrogate decision-makers exists, or judicial involvement is anticipated. (Dastidar and Odden 2011, p. 30)

Art therapy can be especially useful in these gray areas of determination. Both structured and unstructured art therapy directives can be used as an informal assessment tool to measure capacity, since much of art making requires decision making skills utilizing executive functions such as planning and judgment skills, anticipation of consequences, and organizing and prioritizing information, as well as skills used in problem solving. Similarly, the ACLS screens for these same areas of functioning, suggesting that art therapists may also find it useful to use modified art therapy directives to informally assess cognitive capacity.

## Recommendations for support and surrogacy

When an informal art therapy assessment suggests an individual is in need of support or surrogacy in order to maintain quality of life, the art therapist should make a recommendation to a psychologist or psychiatrist for a more formal assessment. The assessment should also include an inquiry into what type of support systems are available, in particular the availability of family support, since cognitively impaired clients are better prepared for increased levels of dependency when surrounded by family and community resource services (Hunt 2003).

Specifically, the most effective approach is structured, team-based support that provides opportunities for autonomous functioning while simultaneously providing increased support as cognition diminishes. Sadly, many clients with impaired cognition lack close family support and, even worse, tend to isolate themselves as their faculties deteriorate (Holmén, Ericsson, and Winblad 2000; Love *et al.* 2011). Therefore, clinicians working with these populations should be sure clients are connected with social service providers to help facilitate a well-integrated, team-based approach to support.

———————————————

Audrey's case examples the importance of this type of integrated support that is imperative for continuity of care in the later stages of dementia. Audrey was fortunate to have a dedicated husband and the financial means to engage support services for herself and for respite for her husband. Her support team included two main non-family caregivers, both of whom were certified in areas of healthcare and had extensive experience with patients with dementia. One caregiver helped Audrey from 10am to 6pm each weekday. She handled toilet issues, walking, feeding, bathing, and provided general companionship. Another caregiver helped on an as needed basis in the evenings. Together, they occasionally provided around-the-clock support if her husband needed to be away. When Gary was home, he cooked supper, helped Audrey with toileting and bathing, got her to bed with a nightly diaper change at 4am, bathed, dressed, combed her hair, made breakfast, and prepared her for the caretaker's arrival. Most importantly, the caregivers provided him with relief during the day so that he could attend to general management of the household and finances.

Clearly, Audrey's daily care required a high level of coordniation, commitment, and responsibility. A basic tenet of her husband's care program for Audrey was to maintain a comforting and constant routine in a familiar setting. When asked if he had ever had second thoughts about continuing to care for Audrey at home, Gary replied:

> It sometimes crosses my mind when I reflect on the inherent confinement her condition imposes on me… [Audrey] is a compliant patient whose gradual if relentless decline has given me time to adjust to her increasing needs. Despite the constant worsening I

can still say I enjoy helping her. The presence of her
art and 50 years of mostly great memories underpin
my commitment to being with her and supporting
her as long as we have the means.

Clearly, dedicated caregivers and empathic surrogates provide
the most effective care for individuals with advanced cognitive
impairments. Aside from considering her best needs, in order
for Audrey's husband to be an effective surrogate, he needed
to truly understand and embrace Audrey's core values during
the decision making process. As art therapists, we may not have
the capacity to offer this level of support to our clients, but
we may find ourselves in a position to best utilize diagnostic
material to expedite intervention, particularly in consideration
of our ethical responsibility as clinicians. Building a therapeutic
relationship based on core values, with consideration of a
client's self-worth, dignity, and right to confidentiality will
assist in ethical clinical practice with cognitively impaired
individuals. Additionally, the art process can help to expedite
intervention, increase the capacity for decision making and
level of engagement, and improve the general quality of life for
these individuals.

---

CHAPTER 3

# Electronic Transmission of Confidential Information and Artwork

## Introduction

Clinical work as a practicing art therapist or art therapy intern often requires communicating confidential information about clients with other clinicians, staff, educators, or peers. As electronic transmission of data continues to become the standard mode of information exchange, many art therapists will use this form of communication. This chapter will clarify some of the general ethical and legal guidelines for electronic transmission of artwork and confidential data in educational and clinical settings.

As defined by the Privacy Rule of The Health Insurance Portability and Accountability Act of 1996 (HIPAA), confidential or protected health information (PHI) includes any documentation of information collected pertaining to a client's mental health progress or treatment. For art therapists, this would include any information about a client, such as progress notes, history, photographs or videos, evaluations, diagnostic material, and client artwork in either original or digital format. Because artwork is created in sessions for both diagnostic and therapeutic purposes, it may be considered PHI in that it can contain identifying information. For art therapy students and interns, client artwork, process notes, case studies or presentations, journal entries, notes on client histories, research papers, journals, personal notes, or any other material for school assignments that relate to contact with clients may contain PHI.

## Identifying information

According to HIPAA, identifying information includes, but is not limited to, the client's name, address, date of birth, institutional facility where the client is being seen, names of family members, and any other personal description or information that might otherwise identify a person (HIPAA 1996). For example, if a person has a specific and unusual identity or profession, such as a celebrity or a notorious criminal history, or an usual medical condition, disability, or personal circumstance, this may not be revealed as the information might clearly identify them.

For art therapists, identifying information can also be found on artwork produced in sessions. Client signatures, personal tags, labeling of family members, addresses, and any other specific or personal, visual, or written reference can be considered identifying information. Additionally, though not considered identifying information as such, documenting or sharing the personal expression of intimate feelings and experience in artwork can be considered a breach of a client's privacy (Haeseler 1992; Hammond and Gantt 1998; Moriya 2006). Directives used in many art therapy evaluations may encourage clients to disclose personal information in the art content as part of the diagnostic art process, so clinicians should consider whether this content can identify clients when preparing to electronically transmit or take digital images of artwork made for evaluation purposes (Alders *et al.* 2011; ATCB 2011; Kapitan 2007).

## CASE SCENARIO

A graduate art therapy student attending class one day was surprised to recognize her close friend's artwork as it appeared onscreen during the professor's lecture. Though the professor used all measures of de-identifying the client's information, the student was still able to recognize elements in her friend's artwork, based on her familiarity with her friend's unusual artistic style. After much consideration and deliberation, the student informed the professor that she was able to identify the client by her artwork because of their close relationship. With this new information, the professor removed that particular client's art from any future lecture material, so as not to further compromise the client's confidentiality.

Art therapists have an especially difficult time ensuring that artwork has been properly de-identified. Information such as a date of birth or town of origin can be removed from artwork, but it can be difficult to tell what other kinds of visual content in art could be potentially identifiable. Furthermore, the small and insular nature of the art therapy profession can increase the possibility of client recognition, even with the most diligent efforts for concealment of identity. In the case of accidental disclosure, it is the ethical responsibility of the person who realizes the breach to inform the clinician, so that dissemination of information can be minimized.

## De-identified information

The HIPAA Privacy Rule states that information can only be exchanged with appropriate release forms and between specific parties on a need-to-know basis that is for the benefit of the

client's treatment (HIPAA 1996, 45 CFR § 164.514). Exceptions
to this would be a need to disclose PHI to law enforcement or
for the purposes of mandated reporting or in the event of a
serious public health risk (HIPAA 1996, 45 CFR § 164.512).
If, however, information is de-identified, it can be used under
certain circumstances for education, research, or demographic
statistics without consent (HIPAA 1996, 45 CFR § 164.502).
The Privacy Rule lists 18 identifiers which must be eliminated
or concealed in order for information to be de-identified. These
identifiers include a person's name, address, social security
number, full face photographs or comparable images, and
birthdate, among other identifying information. Even so, there is
increasing evidence that de-identified information can be easily
re-identified with the plethora of auxiliary information available
from data mining applications in internet usage (Porter 2008).

## Secure transmission

The Privacy Rule also states that confidential information can
only be transmitted electronically under certain conditions that
ensure that diligent attempts are made to protect security of client
information. When confidential information is electronically
transmitted, HIPAA guidelines, as well as any confidentiality
guidelines outlined by an employer or internship placement,
must be observed in order to maintain client confidentiality. In
addition, HIPAA guidelines state that if there is a conflict of
guidelines between state and federal guidelines, state guidelines
will defer to federal guidelines (HIPAA 1996). Additionally, if
one entity has more specific guidelines without conflict, then
the more specific guidelines should be followed.

The AATA also refers to guidelines for electronic
transmission of data, stating that art therapists who choose to
use this mode of transmission are governed by the association's
ethical principles. In addition, AATA also advises that art
therapists should be aware of the risks associated with this kind

of transmission, and that art therapists make themselves aware of any state laws that govern electronic transmissions in their state of practice (AATA 2011, paragraph 14.0). While these guidelines are not specific, this does not mean that art therapists should refrain from electronic transmission. Avoidance would be unrealistic and short of impossible, given the prevalence of digital transmission in the daily usage of clinical communication. Instead, in these vague areas, ethical responsibility dictates both adequate training in digital technology as well as an awareness of federal, state, institutional, and related professional field guidelines for using this type of communication.

The Privacy Rule requires that email servers be encrypted, or some equivalent measure,to ensure that data is being transmitted privately (HIPAA 1996, §164.312). Encryption is the process of transforming digital data using an algorithm to make it unreadable to any system except those possessing a special key. Secure servers use a certificate exchange for identification and encryption to transfer information. Users can send confidential information in a manner that makes it difficult to be intercepted, tracked, or mined. In order to make sure your server is secure, look for the encrypted symbol in the address bar (https://) before the web address, which ensures that a webpage is encrypted. Because the complex transmission of encryption slows down service, some providers do not use it. Checking with your internet service provider or ITS (information technologies services) department whether a site is encrypted is a good policy, if you are unsure.

Just because a particular page or application in a program is encrypted does not mean all applications on the site are secure. For example, log on pages in an email program may be protected but any content that you transmit in an email may not be. Moving back and forth between applications in a mail server or transmitting over portions of an unsecured network can create potential breaches, so, even with encrypted servers, there are potential security risks. Free applications and free email servers often contain program applications that utilize data mining, keystroke logging, and other forms of digital tracking technology, so, in general, it is prudent to avoid any source of free servers and applications of any kind when transmitting confidential data. Even within closed and encrypted digital transmission systems, wireless devices such as laptops, smart phones, Bluetooth devices, PDAs, wireless printers, and wireless copiers can present a security risk, as they can operate on portions of unsecured networks. Ethically and legally, it is the responsibility of the art therapist to take diligent and informed precautions to ensure the confidentiality of clients' private information.

## Minimizing disclosure in digital transmission

As electronic media and storage devices constantly evolve in sophistication, accessibility, and ease of use, there will be an ever-increasing number of ways to capture, store, and transmit digital information. At present, electronic transmission of confidential data includes, but is not limited to, sending confidential information in an email, sending an attachment of a confidential document in an email, sending digital photos of artwork made by clients to yourself or others, and transferring confidential data on to your home or work computer hard drive, cloud storage, USB stick, portable drive, or any other storage device. Additionally, even with the appropriate consent, one of the most difficult aspects of digital transmission data security is that the sender may never be aware that their information has been inadvertently released or captured by unauthorized sources.

Because it is not always possible to tell if PHI has been accidently released, precautions should be taken to minimize disclosure by either de-identifying data before transmission or providing means to recapture data, if misdirected. For example, at minimum, emails should always have a signature attachment in the event they are misdirected. Emails that contain digital images of client artwork should also contain the same kind of signature. The following is a generic sample signature, but it is advised that you refer to your institutional guidelines or legal advisors for more specific wording:

> Notice: The information and/or attachment contained in this electronic message is confidential and is, or may be, protected by the therapist-client privilege and/or other applicable protections from disclosure. If the reader of this message is not the intended recipient, you are hereby notified that any use, dissemination, distribution, or reproduction of this communication is strictly prohibited. If you have received this communication in error, please delete the email from your computer, destroy all copies, and immediately notify my office address, phone number, or email noted above. Thank you.

In the same way, precautions should be taken when storing and deleting files, to minimize unwanted confidential data disclosure. Empty the recycle bin of the computer and clear the temporary internet file folder in the internet browser regularly and frequently. If, for any reason, you are storing a copy of files that contain client information on a hard drive, encrypt the folder which contains the information. Delete the stored files as deemed appropriate.

Keep in mind that files and folders that you delete from your computer are not completely deleted but rather, they are hidden by removing the reference of the file from the file system table of your hard disk. The files can still be retrieved at a later date. Generally, this is not a problem in institutional settings, as IT departments will generally clear hard drives once an employee leaves, but for practitioners using home or office settings, the burden of responsibility is greater. Use a disk erase program or reformat the hard drive to completely remove sensitive files or folders containing client information from your system, which should be done on a regular basis. Because there is always a chance that devices could get lost or stolen and become a potential hazard, avoid, if possible, copying client data to your personal laptop from your work computer, and take care to secure and minimize transport of any portable devices such as external hard disks or storage devices such as CDs, DVDs, etc. For home or office data storage, data should be transferred to an external portable drive, removed after use, and locked in a secure file cabinet for storage, in the same manner in which written files would be protected (Brandoff and Lombardi 2012).

## Minimizing disclosure of confidential information in digital transmission

- Use secured, encrypted servers. Do not use free email servers.

- Do not open sensitive documents in online viewing programs.

- Do not use instant messaging programs to send confidential information.

- Avoid transferring files to your personal computer, USB sticks, CDs, or other storage devices. Use an external drive that is removed and secured in a locked location.

- Delete unnecessary files and empty your trash bin. Delete temporary internet files.

- Periodically erase your hard drive or use a disk erase program.

- Remember to remove identifying information from digital images of artwork BEFORE you photograph artwork.

## Consideration of client rights with artwork

Depending on the guidelines of the institution, client artwork is either considered the property of the client or the client's case file (Moriya 2006; Spaniol 1994). Client artwork cannot be photographed, copied, shared, distributed, disseminated, or used in any kind of research, professional or educational paper, or presentation without permission. With the ease and accessibility of scanners, cameras, and electronic transfer methods, it is easy to forget that any digital image of an original piece of artwork carries the same usage restrictions as those that are applicable to an original piece of art.

Digital images of artwork (from a digital camera, scanner, or cell phone) can only be taken if there is a signed consent form (HIPAA 1996). Even with proper consent, it is good practice to cover identifying information before you take the photo, in the event that the digital file is inadvertently released, lost, or misplaced. With the availability of camera applications on cell phones in particular, it is important to remember that without proper consent, it is a violation of client rights to take digital images of their artwork, even with client names obscured, because there is still a possibility of identification.

Even with a signed consent form, digital images should not be transmitted over unsecured servers or networks. This means, for example, that you cannot take a camera phone picture and then email it to yourself or another party over a non-encrypted server. Many institutions have banned the use of cell phones because of the misuse of cell phone cameras that have violated patient rights (Silas 2011). In addition to the patient's violation, camera phones make it easier to disseminate an inappropriately procured image easily to the internet, directly from the phone (Kapitan 2007). Even with proper consent, using camera phones to photograph artwork is risky, especially when used to store or transfer the digital images. Since it is not always possible to tell if your mobile device is using a secure network, it is advisable not to send images in this manner. Use only a digital camera and transfer digital images via USB cable to a storage device. When you are finished using the image, delete the files and use a disk erase program to ensure complete removal of the files.

If you do not have signed consent forms to photograph or copy art and you need to refer to a client's artwork for supervision or other educational purposes, the best way to maintain confidentiality is to create a facsimile of the artwork that has been produced. To the best of your ability, recreate the piece of art as you observed it, keeping in mind, of course, to omit any identifying content or information. The facsimile can only be used for educational purposes and cannot be reproduced for any other intention. As an educational tool, facsimiles can enhance a visual description of the art and can aid in the supervision process while maintaining a client's right to anonymity.

Because electronic imagery is so easily captured and transmitted in today's digital world, there seems to come with it a diminished consideration for privacy, along with an increase in uncertainty concerning personal and professional boundaries. Just because digital images are easily acquired, it does not therefore imply they can be reproduced, reused, and transferred without permission (ATCB 2011, 3.2.3). Perhaps because a digital image seems to have less physical substance in its digital format than original art, there is less consideration of the ethical and legal impact for students and professionals to regularly store client artwork on their personal laptops and camera phones. Yet, it is unlikely that they would consider constantly carrying around original client artwork on their person. This phenomenon creates a whole new area of ethical consideration for client privacy (Orr 2012). Often, asking a supervisee to consider how they would feel if they created a piece of artwork in session with an art therapist, only to discover that it was captured and stored on their therapist's cell phone alongside photos of their therapist's family or pets, will rekindle a strengthening of therapist-client boundaries in the context of the storage of digital images of client art.

## Art therapy over the internet

A growing trend amongst students, clinicians, and therapists involves using internet video applications to communicate information about clients, engage in distance supervision, and even have virtual therapy sessions when a face-to-face meeting is not possible. This trend is on the rise, in part because of a growing need for experienced supervisors in the expanding field of art therapy, as well as more stringent requirements for state licensing requirements (Brandoff and Lombardi 2012). There are several forms of visual and audio digital communication that take place over the internet rather than a standard land line, many of which are appealing because they are provided as free services. As with free email servers however, free video conferencing programs may not securely transmit digital content, and it is the ethical responsibility of the clinician to make this determination before engaging in any kind of telemental health services (American Telemedicine Association 2009).

Utilizing internet video applications requires a good deal of preliminary consideration in order to minimize potential breaches of ethical issues in the therapeutic and supervisory process. For example, using internet video applications makes it easier to create fraudulent identities. There is also a lack of awareness of compromised confidentiality because of the limited scope of the video camera. It might not always be possible for a participant to see unauthorized individuals entering a video conference setting or know if a room is secure. The American Telemedicine Association (2009) recommends that prior to the start of a telemental health session, the video camera should pan the room and request that individuals present at both locations announce themselves in an attempt to convey a private setting. Moreover, while video conferencing can provide options for individuals in rural, remote, and otherwise inaccessible locations to receive supervision or psychotherapy services, practitioners must be sure to abide by all regulatory authorities in all locations, if the conferences cross state or federal lines.

Art therapy over the internet poses additional considerations for best practices. The interactive quality and tactile nature of the art medium between therapist and client is inherently lost in a video session. Subtle non-verbal body and facial cues can be missed and, in general, there is a lack of the intimacy of real life interaction which may compromise some of the didactic aspects of an art therapy session that involves, for example, teaching a client how to use a new kind of material or technique. This educational component of art therapy can not only increase a client's capacity for artistic expression but also strengthen the therapeutic relationship. Clearly, this aspect of art therapy will be diminished greatly over the internet (Brandoff and Lombardi 2012).

Art therapists also consider the preparation of the art therapy room a large part of the therapeutic process. Easy access to materials, adequate lighting, and an inviting environment can add to the enhancement of the expressive process. Just because video conferencing does not permit access to the therapist's environment, it is still important to create a visually pleasing backdrop for a video session. The American Telemedicine Association (2009) outlines specific guidelines for backgrounds and lighting, suggesting full spectrum, florescent, or daylight which illuminates the practitioner's face and hands. Backgrounds should be simple and clutter free, so as not to be distracting or personally revealing in any way that would distract from the professional focus of the session.

## Final considerations

Distance art therapy and supervision can be an excellent way to make art therapy accessible to those who are homebound, and it is a good option for people that have apprehension or anxiety about seeking therapy. Most importantly, it can help smooth transitions when clients change location quickly and need time to locate a new therapist. When considering whether or not telemental health services are therapeutically warranted, determine first if the situation will most likely be a temporary or long term approach. Review the client's therapeutic goals and needs. Do goals include increasing socialization skills, trust, or intimacy? If so, long-term use of video sessions may not address these issues. Be sure you can provide a secure setting with adequate equipment, internet connection, and screen or monitor resolution, and be sure your client can provide the same. Proper equipment will enhance the visual quality of the video sessions. Discuss with your client, ahead of time, both the benefits and the disadvantages involved in internet therapy or supervision. Be sure to familiarize yourself with state and federal guidelines for the secure transmission of digital data and create a plan for securely storing and deleting any digital files from video sessions.

# CHAPTER 4

# Exchanging Gifts in Art Therapy

## Introduction

Although the topic of giving and receiving gifts in therapy is often discussed, little is written about the topic in ethical guidelines. Similarly, there is a paucity of information on either the benefits or harm of exchanging gifts in a therapeutic context. The scant research that is available is generally based on self-reported information from therapists about their experiences with gifts in therapy, both given and received. According to the data, while some therapists never accept gifts of any sort, most will accept some gifts, depending on the size, value, function, and type of gift, as well as the perceived motivations of the client in giving it (Gerson and Fox 1999; Knapp and VandeCreek 2006; Spandler *et al.* 2000). Though anecdotal experience seems to suggest that a present from a therapist can evoke a strong response in a client, little is written about receiving a gift from the client's perspective, suggestive of a need for more research in this area.

## The complexities of giving and receiving

Whether a gift is given or received, accepted or rejected, most therapists agree that the client's treatment goals, in conjunction with the timing in the course of treatment when the gift exchange occurs, should be carefully considered, and at times openly discussed as part of the treatment process (Spandler *et al.* 2000). A gift given by a therapist to a client struggling with attachment issues may serve as a kind of transitional object to help decrease anxiety during periods of separation in treatment or as an aid in the termination process (Levin and Wermer 1966; Zur 2007). During a holiday break, for example, one therapist described giving an anxious child client in foster care a small pocket calendar with the time of the client's return to treatment clearly marked. Some therapists describe using small tokens, certificates, or mementos to acknowledge a client's successful completion of a cycle of treatment. A tangible keepsake such as this, given by the therapist, can be particularly effective with concrete populations or with children that have difficulty internalizing successful milestones, much in the same way that accumulating stars on a behavioral chart or measuring physical growth with marks on a wall can, over time, help a child to visualize progress (Levin and Wermer 1966). Similarly, a small gift that symbolically represents some aspect of treatment, such as a little box to place wishes and affirmations or a journal for writing down thoughts and feelings presented to a client at the end of treatment, can serve as a kind of transitional object to assist the client in their journey from the protective therapeutic environment into the real world (Rutan and Stone 2001). The therapeutic success of these types of exchanges seems to lie in the relationship of the gift to some symbolic aspect of treatment.

Giving and receiving gifts remains a complex topic in treatment with a manner of response that is situationally dependent (Knox 2008; Koocher and Keith-Spiefel 1998). For instance, if a client gives a gift to a therapist as an expression of appreciation for the therapeutic rapport, a refusal of this gift might have an adverse effect on the therapeutic relationship

(Herlihy and Corey 1997). Some clients with histories of deprivation will exhibit excessive greed and impulsivity, taking art supplies or even stealing from a therapist during sessions. In this case, a client that is able to offer a gift may demonstrate a genuine and improved altruistic capacity to give to others (Levin and Wermer 1966; Stein 1965). On the other hand, rejecting a gift given in this context may suggest to the client that his expanding sense of generosity is not recognized by the therapist.

Most therapists agree that ethnic and cultural norms may also dictate that a therapist accept a gift, if it is not of great monetary value or if it seems that refusal might be considered insulting to a client (Koocher and Keith-Speigel 1998). However, some institutional, state, and federal guidelines, particularly within the judicial system, clearly state that accepting gifts of large monetary value may influence treatment in a negative way, thus crossing ethical and perhaps even legal boundaries. These guidelines are generally implemented to reduce the possibility of collusion in illegal or unethical activities and minimize bribery and influence on decisional procedures within the institutional setting. In general, any gift that is significant enough, material or otherwise, to create a feeling of obligation or manipulate professional judgment should be refused.

While receiving gifts can be complicated, giving gifts to clients seems to give rise to even more complex ethical considerations. A thoughtful gift from a therapist can have the benefit of strengthening the therapeutic relationship and creating a more nurturing therapeutic environment. At the same time, even when well intended, giving a gift to a client can also increase anxiety, expectations, disappointment, and fears about obligatory reciprocation (Levin and Wermer 1966). Gift-giving in child populations or in group therapy settings can often stir up feelings of rivalry and competition for attention, increasing tensions amongst clients, especially if the therapist gives different gifts to each client. Yet, giving the same gift to all group members can make some members feel they are not perceived as a unique and individual member. In this instance, they may chose to not accept the gift at all, creating uneasiness and tension in the group. Even when a well considered gift is presented to a client, they may still chose to reject it, usually signifying an expression of passive or blatant hostility, a rejection of one's own identity, or fear of conditional indebtedness to the therapist or the treatment process (Levin and Wermer 1966).

## Artwork as a gift in treatment

Though the ATCB (2011, § 3.4.7) refers specifically to gift-giving in its code of ethics, the guidelines do not support or dissuade a therapist from accepting gifts. Rather, the guidelines acknowledge the complexity of the dilemma and encourage the therapist to consider the motivations for both giving and receiving, the monetary value of the gift, and the reasons why a client may want to give, taking into consideration cultural and societal norms. The guidelines do not address the concept of giving artwork as a gift, which is inherently present in the art therapy setting and presents even more challenging considerations. If general consensus among clinicians and ethical guiding principles recommend the consideration of the material and symbolic significance of a gift, how does one determine the material value and emotional significance of artwork produced in a therapeutic session? Furthermore, would the value of the art be different if it was not produced in session?

Anecdotally, most art therapists agree that artwork produced in session has a different relational value than work produced outside of sessions. One of the guiding principles in the use of art as psychotherapy is that the art serves as an externalized documentation of the therapeutic process (Landgarten 1981; Malchiodi 1998). With this understanding, acceptance of a gift of art made in a session from a client is then denying the client the option to keep that record of the therapeutic process. In the moment, offering the gift to the therapist may be a genuine expression of gratitude, but this may change over time. As treatment progresses and insight increases, the client may realize that the artwork could have served as a measure of this progress. For this reason, accepting client art made in sessions should always be discussed openly as part of the therapeutic process, allowing the therapist to help the client anticipate the possible negative consequences of giving the work away.

## CASE SCENARIO

An art therapist working in an adult inpatient psychiatric facility ran a weekly art therapy group focusing on women's issues. One group member, a woman in her late thirties with a long history of sexual abuse, had for the first time disclosed the abuse in one particular group, being inspired by a particularly compelling directive. As a token of gratitude to the art therapist, the client offered the work as a gift and the therapist, not wanting to offend the client, gratefully accepted. Several weeks later as she prepared for discharge, during one of the art therapy groups, the client made a reference to the piece of art she had made and subsequently given to the art therapist, remarking how the piece had come to represent an important moment in her healing process. In response, on the day of the client's discharge, the art therapist carefully wrapped and presented the artwork back to the client as a parting gift. The client seemed very relieved and grateful, only admitting then that she wished she had not given the art away in the first place but felt uncomfortable asking for it back.

In this case, the art therapist was sensitive to both the client's different needs at various points in the therapeutic process. When the client first offered the art, following a powerful and cathartic disclosure, had the therapist not accepted the gift of art, the client may have felt a keen sense of rejection, which may have influenced her subsequent ability to be able to wholly participate in treatment. Abuse victims often feel damaged and unworthy, further enforcing the secrecy and shame of the abuse. The artwork represented the disclosure of these events and also a projection of the client (Pifalo 2002). Rejecting this, would in effect, be symbolically rejecting the client, reinforcing her feelings of being damaged or unworthy. Later, as the client's treatment progressed, and she seemed more comfortable with the therapeutic process and her growing sense of self, the value of the moment of initial disclosure documented in her artwork became evident to the client. Keeping a connection to the artwork and the valuable process it represented was important. Recognizing this, the art therapist returned the artwork.

---

Anticipating and addressing these possible consequences when the client first offers the artwork can not only enhance the therapeutic process but also reduce the incidents of awkwardness. Similarly, with other populations, such as impulse ridden clients, individuals with pervasive developmental disorders, and some children and adolescents, it is important to discuss possible regret and feelings of loss after giving away art, before making a decision to do so. For some traumatized and abused populations, giving the artwork away may symbolize a recurrent pattern of having to surrender some part of themselves in order to receive acceptance, love, or attention. Individuals that have difficulty with self care may be unable to keep something for themselves and should be encouraged to do so.

Still, there may be instances when giving away art made in sessions can be therapeutically productive. Clients may find it easier to give away a functional object, rather than a deeply personal and provocative piece, in defense of possible rejection by the receiver (Henley 2002). Additionally, the client can benefit from the appreciation and usefulness of the gift when it is received. Art therapists working in correctional facilities have described the significance of giving functional gifts or hand-made cards as a means of staying connected with family and loved ones during the isolation of incarceration. Some traumatized individuals may have a strong need to give their art to a therapist. Perhaps because of the powerful symbolic content in art, a client may need to give away this art because the content is intolerable or too difficult to accept themselves, hoping to see, instead, how the therapist will manage the feelings symbolically expressed in the work.

## CASE SCENARIO

An art therapist, working in a community based program with adults with chronic mental illness, described an intriguing painting that was given to her by a male client diagnosed with paranoid schizophrenia. She described this client as having difficulty with social interactions and difficult to engage on an interpersonal level, so she was touched by his gesture of giving. A prolific painter, the client had made the piece outside of therapy, in his home, but the piece was typical of much of the work he had produced in group sessions, expressing idiosyncratic and peculiar imagery reflecting the content of his bizarre delusions. On a personal level, the art therapist found the work extremely appealing both conceptually and formally, as a practicing artist herself, in his bold use of line and provocative figurative schema. Though she admitted that she would have enjoyed taking the piece home, the art therapist instead hung the work in her office, in an attempt to maintain professional and personal boundaries. In offering the painting, the art therapist felt that it was important to accept the work, because of the client's difficulty engaging in the therapeutic relationship as well as her general experience of emotional impoverishment, neediness, and narcissistic preoccupation with this population in general which often made it difficult for them to give to others. The art therapist felt comfortable accepting the work as it was created outside of the therapeutic session and did not seem to represent a documentation of any particular event in treatment. Rather, because the client was a prolific painter, the painting carried less significance than if making the gift had been an infrequent production. In her opinion, giving the painting seemed to be a statement of his growth in the program as well as an attempt to acknowledge the therapeutic relationship and refusing it, the art therapist believed, might cause damage to the clinical relationship.

## Art therapy directives and gifts

To assist in the exploration of the possible benefits and risk of giving and receiving gifts, art therapy directives can also be created specifically around the concept of giving away the art. For example, asking clients to create something that they will give away or exchange can address both concepts of giving and receiving, and will instinctively alter the approach to the content of the art. These kinds of directives can be especially helpful around holidays and other events that generally include some form of gift-giving ritual. At the same time, these directive may heighten feelings of loss and disappointment, so art therapists should consider the needs of their specific population at the outset. Sometimes, a joint art making directive which allows for both therapist and client to participate in the art making process on a shared canvas or paper can diffuse some of the feelings of disappointment and obligation that might otherwise occur in a more traditional gift exchange. For example, creating a joint scribble drawing together or using a printmaking technique to create multiple images that can be shared can also diffuse feelings of loss.

Giving and receiving artwork as a gift in therapy is a complicated topic for art therapists. No doubt, gift-giving holds unconscious communications between the giver and receiver, and when this is complicated by the unconscious expression of artwork made in treatment, there is great possibility of misinterpretation. Careful consideration of both the content of the art and the context of when the art was made should be explored, preferably with the client, to ensure anticipatory responses to the gift exchange experience.

### Considerations for gift exchange in art therapy:

- For non-art gifts, consider the material value of the item.
- For artwork made in sessions, consider the content of the art as well as the context in which it was created.
- Help clients to anticipate benefit and risks of giving away art made in sessions.
- Explore the client's motivation to give a gift.
- Be sensitive to the ethnic and cultural norms of gift-giving.
- Familiarize yourself with institutional, professional, and legal guidelines about gift exchange with clients.
- Identify all possible outcomes that may affect the therapeutic relationship when giving or receiving a gift.
- When in doubt, seek guidance from a trusted supervisor, mentor, or colleague.

# CHAPTER 5

# Touch and the Therapeutic Art Process

## A history of conflict about touch in therapy

A squeeze of the shoulder, a brief tap on the forearm, or steady, guiding hands to help manipulate a hefty slab of clay can express so much beyond what words can say. It is clear why sexualized touch is not appropriate in the clinical setting, but it is not so easy to determine if there is value or harm in non-erotic touch in therapy. Clinicians are divided about the use of touch in the therapeutic relationship and trends shift over time within the context of changing cultural norms (Strozier, Krizek, and Sale 2003).

The notion of touching clients first became widely popular in the 1960s, following a wave of alternative approaches to traditional psychoanalytically based treatment (Lowenberg, Dolgoff, and Harrington 2004). Decades earlier, touch was introduced by Sigmund Freud in his early work with hypnosis and regression, but not long afterward, Freud abandoned the idea of incorporating touch, feeling that it complicated the concept of transference (Strozier *et al.* 2003). In his early work, Freud described touching his clients on the forehead or clasping their heads between his hands in order to bring unconscious material to the surface and expedite the hypnotic process (Bartole 2011). Similarly, psychoanalyst Sandor Ferenczi felt that not touching clients made the therapist seem aloof and distant. In particular, for those clients who had experienced trauma, withholding touch from a client only recapitulated the trauma. Ferenczi believed that touch embodied an empathic approach to treatment (Strozier *et al.* 2003). Still, most therapists at the time believed that physical contact with clients was not an integral part of psychotherapy. This shift to a more remote style of psychoanalytic therapy set the tone for a continued history of conflict and dispute about the value of touch in clinical treatment.

## The negative implications of touch

Today, some therapists are still leery of any kind of touch at all in a therapeutic environment, fearing that it might be misconstrued and lead to more sexualized contact, especially if it occurs regularly and the client and therapist are matched in terms of sexual orientation (Lowenberg *et al.* 2004). Research on the impact of touch in therapy is inconclusive, making it difficult for therapists to have a decisive opinion on the topic (Lowenberg *et al.* 2004) and thereby simply avoid the issue. This avoidance is only exacerbated by the lack of inclusion of the subject in educational settings and supervision (Burkholder *et al.* 2010). Additionally, clients have different needs, and in fragile states can easily misinterpret the most well-intended non-sexual touch, such as a hug or pat on the back, especially when the client has a history of sexual abuse (Swade, Bayne, and Horton 2006). For many therapists, in an age of copious lawsuits and malpractice accusations, the possibility of misinterpretation of a physical gesture is professionally threatening (Strozier *et al.* 2003). This atmosphere may also inhibit therapists from spontaneously responding with a touch or other empathic physical gesture out of fear of legal reprisal.

A common question in supervision is whether or not to hug clients, especially when a client is visibly distraught or when they ask for or initiate a hug. Most therapists feel that hugging a client is rarely acceptable, and that anything more than a handshake would be less than appropriate (Pope, Tabachnik, and Keith-Spiegel 1987; Stenzel and Rupert 2004). When addressed in supervision, both students and practicing clinicians will sheepishly report that they hugged a client, while admitting that some part of the physical interaction was uncomfortable, either because it invited later breaches of physical boundaries by the client or it violated a level of physical comfort on the part of the clinician. In either case, clinicians' discomfort suggests that therapeutic value was overshadowed by some kind of violation of personal and physical boundaries. Clincians still sometimes feel torn, wanting to respond in a genuine manner, but at a loss as to how to do so without physical contact. While nothing is a good substitute for physical touch, sometimes certain non-physical gestures can convey a sense of empathy and consideration. Maintaining visual contact by holding a client's gaze, leaning in or moving physically closer to a client can imply a sense of undivided attention and authentic concern without physical contact.

In general, most clients respond positively to the idea of therapists touching them in a non-sexual way, as with a touch on the hand or arm, or occasionally a brief hug (Burkholder *et al.* 2010). One has to only do a brief search of the internet to see numerous anonymous posts from individuals in treatment anguishing about whether or not to request some kind of non-sexual physical contact from a therapist. While these needs may be genuinely expressed from clients, symbolically or literally, it does not mean that non-sexual touch is therapeutically warranted. Yet other clients, in particular those with histories of sexual trauma or paranoia, can have a very different response. Some clients may respond to touch by regressing, feeling offended, enraged, or especially vulnerable (Strozier *et al.* 2003).

When considering the ethical implications of touch in therapy, it is important to reflect on your personal style. Do you tend to touch people frequently outside of your professional relationships? What is your cultural norm with regard to touch?

When do you most like to be touched? When do you least like to be touched? Is the way you touch someone differentiated by gender? By exploring your personal style and interpretation of touch, you will feel more comfortable in setting personal boundaries with clients and offering an alternative when a client requests physical contact (Strozier *et al.* 2003). Leaning forward, making eye contact, and offering genuine concern can oftentimes be an excellent substitute for a hug, without having to violate personal boundaries.

When considering touching a client, one should also keep in mind a client's gender, developmental stage, stage of the therapeutic relationship, treatment goals, and client diagnosis or history. It is also important to consider whether or not a client's gender influences how they are touched. Limited physical touch such as a pat on the arm or back can sometimes have therapeutic value with certain young child populations. However, with adolescents, paranoid, aggressive, delusional, or psychotic clients, any kind of physical contact can easily be misinterpreted as sexualized and should generally be avoided unless extenuating situations, ample experience, available supervision, and clinical indication suggest otherwise. Consider carefully whether or not touching the client will have any kind of beneficial effect and seek the advice of mentors, colleagues, and peers when in doubt about touch in a therapeutic setting (Zur 2007a).

## Touch in art therapy

In addition to these general considerations about the inclusion of touch in therapy, art therapists are presented with additional ethical challenges because of the tactile and interactive nature of the art process. All art materials require some level of physical interaction. Moreover, some therapeutic goals with certain populations may include using certain art materials to decrease tactile defensiveness (Sholt and Gavron 2006), so physical interaction with the material and with the art therapist is likely, if not unavoidable.

Certain materials such as clay and finger paint, which require direct manual manipulation, body movement, and tactile interaction, may elicit strong emotional responses that relate back to early tactile memories that were initially determined through touch (Kearns 2004; Sholt and Gavron 2006). Addressing early touch related experiences through tactile art mediums can allow for a safe and healthy recapitulation of early traumas and losses (Anderson 1995; Rubin 2005). Clients with histories of trauma that use the symbolic process of art materials to reenact aspects of their histories may benefit from a more positive recapitulation of a touch experience, so art therapists must explore how to use touch in a comfortable and clinically appropriate manner. Since certain tactile materials can offer a wider range of kinesthetic exploration with hand-over-hand guidance by an art therapist (Henley 2000), avoiding physical contact altogether may limit the value of the art material and art process.

Physical contact for art therapists is sometimes difficult to circumvent, depending on the population and the materials being used. While working with the blind and visually impaired population using tactile materials such as plaster and clay, it is virtually impossible to avoid physical contact since auditory directions are sometimes inadequate when clients are presented with new materials. Hand-over-hand manipulation and guidance is essential for clients who lack visual cues and with complex materials such as clay (Henley 2000). Similarly, pre-school age children and children or adults with pervasive developmental disorders often respond more positively to hand-over-hand modeling, as they are in a stage of development that responds best to sensory-motor experiences (Piaget and Inhelder 1969). Geriatrics and clients in medical and hospice settings may also require more physical contact to facilitate interactions with materials because of declining physical abilities. Regardless of a client's developmental capacity, touch can be used to model, teach, guide, or reassure a client through a challenging art therapy experience.

Outside of demonstrating art materials, touch may be a useful adjunctive tool in an art therapy session to help certain clients maintain focus. When working with children or populations with impulse control issues, a brief touch may be used to redirect a client, get their attention, or to reinforce an important insight or occurrence in the session. Clients that are reluctant to explore a tactile medium with their fingers, such as charcoal or chalk pastel, may benefit from hand-over-hand demonstrations of regulating pressure in order to broaden the range of expression. Clients that are easily stimulated by tactile or fluid materials such as finger paint or clay may benefit from a tactile cue to stop regressive tendencies.

## CASE SCENARIO

An experienced art therapist described a session with an artistically gifted, middle-aged woman who was specifically addressing her history of severe childhood abuse. The client generally worked in easily controlled materials such as graphite and colored pencil, exhibiting an emotional distance from the content, but the art therapist had been slowly, over time, introducing more fluid art mediums to encourage more interaction with the materials, in the hope of a greater emotional connection with the art content. During one session in particular, while working with tissue paper and a liquid polymer adhesive, the client began experimenting with using the adhesive to make the colors in the tissue paper bleed together. Determined to create this effect, she began to use her hands to manipulate the wet colored paper. Quite suddenly, the client's mood shifted. Her body stiffened and her eyes glazed over and the art therapist suspected something in the physical contact with the art materials triggered a traumatic response from her past. Looking down at her hands, the client said softly, "Oh! I'm sorry they're so dirty. Oh! I'm in trouble…"

The therapist responded gently by saying she was not in trouble, reminding her that getting messy while making artwork was perfectly fine and suggested that they clean her hands. The client remained frozen. Deciding to then assist her, the art therapist, all the while speaking softly to the client, guided her to the sink and gently washed her hands under the water, much in the same way a mother would clean a young child's hands. As the stain on the client's hands lightened under the soap and warm water, she became more responsive, making eye contact and speaking to the art therapist. Soon she was able to complete the hand-washing process herself, continue with her collage piece, and ultimately discuss the experience with the art therapist in relationship to her traumatic history.

In this way, the carefully considered physical touch response of the art therapist enabled the client to have a corrective and more positive experience than she had most likely experienced in her past. Words alone may not have been effective in allowing this client to be released from the paralyzing trauma trigger, nor would it have allowed for such a powerful recapitulation of a positive tactile experience through both the art medium and physical contact with the art therapist.

## Minimizing the misinterpretation of touch

Always, before touching clients, the therapeutic value of any kind of touch should be considered carefully, keeping in mind the client's best interests as well as the therapist's level of experience and competence. Use peer support or supervision when in doubt. Assess the ability of a client to differentiate between various forms of touch based on their developmental levels of functioning and diagnosis.

When working with clients that may be at risk of misunderstanding touch, the art therapist should consider the minimum amount of physical contact that is needed to demonstrate art material techniques. For therapist initiated touch, even though the intent might be clear to the therapist, it may not be interpreted in the same manner by the client (Zur 2007a; Zur 2007b). Generally, demonstrating next to or across from a client, rather than from behind, minimizes unnecessary full body contact. Sitting next to, rather than standing over, a client while making contact, can reduce any perceived power differential when working with clients that have any kind of trauma history. Whenever possible, wear long sleeved shirts and/or art smocks when demonstrating art materials, to minimize skin-to-skin contact which can be stimulating and more easily misconstrued with some client populations.

Sometimes, letting a client know that you may touch them or asking permission before the art material demonstration can easily clarify the intent of touch and communicate the therapist's respect for personal boundaries. For example, a client may ask for assistance with an art material, not realizing it involves touch. The art therapist could say something as simple as, "If you want me to help you carry that slab of clay over to the table, I may need to stand close to you or touch you. If that's not comfortable, I can carry it for you." In this way, the client is made aware beforehand of the possibility of touch, the clear intention, and an option to decline, giving them a sense of empowerment they may not have experienced in past traumatic situations that involved physical contact. While it may not seem to directly address therapeutic goals, these incidental moments in art therapy sessions can have powerful and lasting therapeutic effects, when handled with consideration and forethought.

## When using touch in art therapy:

- Consider the motives for using touch by focusing on the client's goals. Never use touch to gratify personal needs or with sexual intent.

- Explore your own ideas, limitations, and interpretations of various forms of touch.

- Consider the social, ethnic, and cultural implications of touch.

- Consider the timing in treatment when using touch. Therapeutic relationships in the early stages of formation invite greater possibilities for the misinterpretation of touch.

- Consider the history and diagnosis of your client. While certain trauma, paranoid, and impulse ridden populations can benefit from touch in treatment, these populations also present the greatest opportunities for negative responses to touch.

- Ask your client for permission to touch or use hand-over-hand techniques with art materials to impart a sense of respect for their personal physical boundaries.

- Seek supervision or peer support when in doubt.

CHAPTER 6

# Spirituality in Art and Therapy

## Introduction

The concepts of spirituality and religion are often used interchangeably, although their meanings are somewhat different. Spirituality can be defined as a person's connection or conceptual understanding of the notion of God, whereas religion is the actual ritualistic practices that have developed to reflect one's spirituality (Hamdam 2008). Religious practices are often exhibited in a social context with others who share similar beliefs (Gallup and Jones 2000; Hodge 2011). Ethical practice advocates that clinicians support a client's ethnic, cultural, and spiritual belief systems, in part because of the important role of these values in positive treatment outcomes (Barnett and Johnson 2011; Dein 2004; Frame 2000; Kliewer 2004; Sue and Sue 2008). Specifically, a strongly defined sense of spirituality can enhance a client's self identity and create a reliable support system in their religious community (Hodge 2011; Miller 1998).

Many cultures, including Native and Central American, Asian and Afro-Caribbean cultures, ascribe healing as mutually dependent upon religious practice (Koepfer 2000; Tseng and McDermott 1981; Van Hoecke 2006), so it may be difficult, if not unethical, to ignore this spiritual aspect in treatment. Advocacy and support of a client's spirituality in treatment can be demonstrated by assessing, for example, how the ritual of social religious practice might decrease anxiety or provide an additional means of support through the client's religious social community. Certain types of religious rituals, such as prayer and meditation, or a renewed interest in spirituality, can distract clients from negative thoughts and non-productive behaviors, while also assisting clients in creating a sense of closure during times of stress, in particular in the final stages of a terminal illness (Kubler-Ross 1983; Furman 2011). This kind of therapeutic support requires that the therapist be open and curious to learn about how the client's spirituality best serves the client and can be implemented regardless of the therapist's own religious orientation (Tan 2003).

While the integration of healing and religious practice in cultural contexts can be beneficial, care must be taken when integrating spirituality into clinical healing practices. Certain forms of psychotherapy, especially creative arts therapies, are highly dependent on the use of symbolism as part of the healing process, creating a natural proclivity towards blending spirituality and healing (Dow 1986). The merging of these two concepts can simultaneously create enhanced capacities for healing as well as the potential for blurred boundaries, and confusions in scope of practice. Additionally, alternative spiritual beliefs may be in direct conflict with traditional religious practice adding to further confusion in the therapeutic setting (Lori et al. 2009; Plante 2007). At times, personal interest in a particular form of spirituality may inspire a therapist to integrate a particular religious ritual into clinical practice, regardless of the relevance to treatment goals or benefit to the specific patient population. Similarly, professional licensed practitioners without specific theological training are not clerical counselors, and since most graduate psychotherapy and creative arts therapy programs do not include religious counseling training, practice of this nature would reflect a level of incompetence (Plante 2007).

Because art therapy is a blend of intuitive and clinical skill, combined with a deep connection to the artistic and healing process, the field draws many individuals who have a strong connection to alternative and spiritually based practices. It is not uncommon for art therapists to have experimented with various creative arts as well as traditional and non-traditional spiritual practices (earth-based religions and shamanism, for example), as part of a personal growth and healing process. Some art therapists incorporate the aspects of new age or conventional spiritual practices into their art therapy practice, such as combining art therapy with yoga or meditation. On the other hand, some art therapists are acutely aware of the professional stigma often attached to this type of integral practice and avoid the use of any kind of spiritual ideology in clinical work, especially in medical, research, and psychological settings, for fear of diluting their professional validity (Bolen 1979; Koepfer 2000; Plante 2007).

## Client expressed spirituality in art therapy

Art therapists have described spontaneous productions of art with religious content from clients in sessions, in particular with clients who are struggling with significant medical, psychological, and terminal illness (Furman 2011; Koepfer 2000; Zammit 2001). These may be expressed in the form of houses of worship, angels, spirits, gods, goddesses, or other religious iconographic symbols in paintings, drawings, or sculptures. The invasive nature of a severe medical illness or psychological trauma often encourages clients to retreat into more esoteric and spiritual quests in an effort to make sense of inordinate levels of pain and suffering in the material world.

---

## CASE SCENARIO

A 16-year-old client was admitted to an outpatient treatment program for feelings of hopelessness, depression, and suicidal ideation after three of her close friends were simultaneously killed in an automobile accident. In art therapy sessions, she initially created black and white pencil images of isolated figures, often hunched over or curled in a ball. As she began to participate more in treatment and her suicidal ideation decreased, the imagery in her artwork changed dramatically. She began to include multiple interactive figures in active, expansive positions, often with arms outstretched. She stated the figures had magical powers and could make wishes come true. In addition to the figures, she often included other magical imagery and religious icons such as angels, fairies, doves, magic wands, stars, and crosses. In her daily life, she began to take interest in a pantheistic earth-based religion that focused on healing through the elements found in nature.

---

## CASE SCENARIO

A 38-year-old woman with terminal bone cancer, who was self-described as having no religious affiliations, created images of churches and cathedrals in her individual art therapy sessions. She became obsessed with details of the different architectural periods of the cathedrals, regularly bringing reference images and books on the topic into her art therapy sessions. While creating the art, she began to talk about how she envisioned her funeral service and how to begin to prepare her children for her imminent death.

---

## CASE SCENARIO

A 52-year-old woman diagnosed with paranoid schizophrenia in an inpatient psychiatric unit entered the open studio group therapy session, sat down, and placed a small carton of orange juice in front of herself. She was known in the unit to carry juice around with her at all times. She began what appeared to be a realistic drawing of the orange juice container in front of her and then added a bearded male face to the front of the carton, whom she identified as Jesus. When asked to share her work with the group, she stated she was very religious and that Jesus was with her all the time, in her orange juice. In response, the art therapist stated he did not actually see Jesus in the carton the same way the client did. The therapist went on to say that sometimes it might be important for people to keep someone or something close to them and people had different ways of doing that. He then asked the rest of the group members if they had ways to keep important people close to them when they were far away, eliciting a conversation with the entire group.

In all three of these examples, the religious content seemed to serve a productive purpose and did not support self-harm or destructive behavior. In the first case, it appeared that the spiritual and magical content seemed to serve as a way to defend against the overwhelming feelings of loss of control and fear of death. The shocking death of the young girl's peers created the possibility that at any moment, she could die, too. In her response of an expressed wish to die, suicide was at least some form of control, if death was inevitable. Her later choice of a pantheistic earth-centered religion based on predictable seasons and lunar tables, without one omnipotent and seemingly unpredictable God, seemed to help the client feel more in control of her confusing feelings, and ultimately allowed her to cope more effectively. Additionally, the art content which reflected magical thinking, in the form of fairies and other magical creatures, seemed to be a regression to an earlier stage of logic and thinking which temporarily allowed her to cope with her trauma. The figures in her art seemed to have omnipotent powers that could make anything come true, a satisfying feeling in a situation that felt out of control, in much the same way as this kind of faulty logic serves to assist young children in coping with stress and trauma (Roberts 2011).

In the second example, the client also felt out of control in the face of a terminal illness. Though she had no personal religious affiliation, it is not uncommon for individuals in the final stages of life to seek some form of spiritual connection to assist in mitigating the finality of imminent death (Kubler-Ross 1983). For this client though, her interaction with spirituality seemed limited to an intellectual and artistic connection. Her preoccupation with the architectural details seemed to help bind her anxieties about her terminal illness, enough to allow her to talk about the future of her children and her funeral plans.

In the last example, it appeared that the client might either be experiencing visual hallucinations or delusions with religious content, though they did not appear to be having any obvious detrimental effects at the time. The therapist's response did not reinforce the delusional content nor did it shame the client, but rather focused on using spiritual beliefs for coping with the illness, thus opening the discussion to the entire group. Had the client's hallucinations or delusions been more obviously malevolent, the intervention would have been different, focusing more on reality-based thinking and reinforcing personal safety, rather than the religious content.

To some degree, Western medicine has pathologized religious preoccupations in certain forms of mental illness such as schizophrenia and psychotic disorders, with little consideration for the positive effects. In addition to the obvious negative effects of violence in the actions of religious extremists, other seemingly less insidious forms of religious preoccupations and delusions can affect day-to-day functioning and even be harmful to patients (Plante 2007). For example, clients who engage in self-harm and mutilation because they experienced religious command hallucinations rather than being highly spiritual, may be using a psychopathological distortion of spirituality to defend deep-seated feelings of a guilt, a lack of self-worth, or aggression (Kaufman 1939; Suhail and Ghauri 2010).

The art therapist's first task is to try to determine if the client is expressing religious convictions in a benign attempt to cope with their illness, or if the content reflects a more distorted interpretation of spirituality that tends towards self-harm. Oftentimes, observing levels of anxiety when a client is engaged in religious practice can indicate if the practice is causing harm. If the practice seems to increase rather than decrease levels of anxiety, the client may be experiencing command hallucinations that are conflictual or harmful to themselves or others. Also, the presence of religious grandiosity, bizarre, aggressive, or paranormal religious content can help distinguish true spiritual faith from religious delusions (Suhail and Ghauri 2010). For example, a client who insists he is God, as opposed to feeling strongly connected to a god or spirit, may be exhibiting delusional thinking, not religious passion.

## Therapist expressed spirituality in art therapy

In each case scenario presented, the religious affiliation of the art therapist was not relevant, as the focus was on client need and the purpose that spirituality or religious ritual served during stressful times. In this approach, a good deal of spiritual and religious content in art and behavior is addressed in the therapeutic setting, in a way that benefits the client without a blurring of personal and professional boundaries by introducing the therapist's spiritual orientation or beliefs. Additionally, this approach can minimize potential ethical dilemmas when therapists express or integrate their own spiritual beliefs into their client's treatment process (Haldmen 2002).

One of the most obvious conflicts in the blending of spirituality and religion is the issue of dual relationships. As previously mentioned, many art therapists have interests in mind-body therapies and may carry certifications in yoga instruction and spiritual healing practices such as Reiki, Ayurveda, or meditation. Without careful consideration, integrating these disciplines into art therapy practice can present problems of confused boundaries for the client in several ways. Limits of confidentiality, for example, are different for clergy and alternative practitioners than for therapists, who are mandated reporters. As this could create both legal and ethical conundrums (Plante 2007; Swenson, Schneller and Sanders 2009), clients should be well advised of their therapist's multiple orientations prior to the start of treatment or counseling of any kind.

When spiritual and psychotherapy practices are integrated, issues of competency and scope of practice are also a potential risk. An interest or personal vocation in a certain spiritual faith does not make a therapist an expert in that religious tradition (Plante 2007). Some certifications in alternative practice are inconsistent and unregulated, making them suspect with regard to competency. Ethical guidelines state that art therapists should be properly trained and educated before performing any kind of method or procedure, and the application should not exceed the professional scope of practice. With regard to services other than art therapy, the ethical guidelines also clearly state art therapists should not offer these kinds of services without certification or licensing in these areas (ATCB 2011). These guidelines do not, however, address the use of religious ritual or spiritual orientation into art therapy practice and therefore must be considered by the practitioner.

## CASE SCENARIO

An art therapist, with a strong attachment to her Christian faith, worked in a women's shelter in a large urban setting, with clients drawn from a wide variety of cultural and ethnic backgrounds. Most of the clients were victims of domestic violence and participation in art therapy sessions was a mandatory program requirement. Often, when her clients were most distressed and hopeless, she encouraged them to pray together at the end of an art therapy session. Clients from non-Christian faiths began to complain to the shelter's director that the joint prayer made them uncomfortable in sessions, though they understood the therapist was well-intended. The art therapist was surprised when confronted with the client complaints, as her private practice, which she openly advertised as a Christian faith based approach to art therapy, was successful and thriving, with an all Christian clientele.

In this case, the art therapist's private practice clientele were well aware of her Christian orientation and had the option to select her, based on this information, if they so desired. These clients would expect the art therapist to integrate spiritual and healing practices into the sessions as well as look forward to shared views and religious core values. The shelter clients, however, were attending mandatory therapy sessions. To be asked to participate in prayer that may be unfamiliar or different from their own prayer practices may have increased rather than appeased anxiety. Additionally, simply because the approach of prayer was helpful to the therapist in times of stress did not mean it would be for her clients. In a clinical environment, client needs and a high level of tolerance for clients' varying cultural and religious backgrounds is necessary before considering integrating spirituality into therapy practice.

## CASE SCENARIO

A licensed and board certified art therapist with additional licensing as a massage therapist and certification as a Reiki master was contemplating opening a healing arts center. The art therapist wanted to offer individual and group art therapy and other healing arts. Before securing a space, the art therapist consulted an attorney familiar with scope of practice issues for clinicians and therapists using art therapy and massage, bodywork, and healing touch (somatic practices) in her home state, to be sure she was in compliance with competency criteria and that she would be appropriately advertising the services she wanted to offer. In addition, she contacted the licensing bodies for both art therapists and massage therapists in her state. She then consulted an art therapy supervisor for regular supervision. On reflection, she decided to hire a second massage therapist and Reiki master for her art therapy clients who wanted these services. Moreover, the art therapist only practiced Reiki and massage with clients she did not see for art therapy.

In this complicated case example, the art therapist was legally and ethically responsible for conforming to any applicable state or federal regulations regarding all of the practice modalities she wished to provide. In particular, because both massage and Reiki involve touch as part of the healing process, there might be additional regulations for their practice. In some states, even with a certificate, a person may not implement a somatic practice without a license. Some Reiki practitioners simply continue to practice without ever making physical contact with their client. Other practitioners have gotten around this law through a loophole that allows for healing touch or a *laying on of hands*, if it is done in a religious context. Some states allow ordained ministers to practice a touch healing technique. Individuals can then easily obtain ordination as a non-denominational minister, regardless of their personal spiritual orientation, and use it as a way to practice within the confines of the law. Websites today advertise simple methods of obtaining minister ordination specifically for this purpose, often in a matter of hours with little or no fee. Given the spiritual context of somatic arts, it is not necessary to extrapolate further since the seemingly unethical implications of obtaining legal compliance to practice a healing art are quite obvious.

More importantly, the art therapist in this case scenario, after seeking out legal and clinical advice, decided to maintain a clear professional boundary by not confusing her clients by only practicing one modality with them. She was able to offer more options by hiring colleagues trained in other services. Given the added complications for art therapists involving touch and the art process, this seemed, in this case, like a professionally responsible decision.

## Recommendations

When considering the integration of spiritual and psychotherapy healing practices, one of the best ways to reduce confusion, misunderstanding, and client disappointment in treatment, is to be clear prior to the start of treatment about the orientation and scope of the practice and to outline realistic client treatment goals. In the hope of reducing confusion during the treatment process, a significant number of faith based practitioners obtain informed consent from a client that allows the use of spiritually based practices in sessions (Swenson, Schneller, and Sanders 2009). Obtaining a consent form of this nature allows for a natural discussion of what the client may expect in terms of spiritual activities. Similarly, in private practice, explicitly advertising that the therapy is spiritually based will also reduce confusion. When providing services in non-ecumenical settings with high levels of religious diversity, keep in mind the needs of the client and look to increase coping skills that fall within a client's own level of comfort, whether secular or religious. Finally, let religious content be initiated by a client. As in other arenas of treatment, client-driven initiatives will allow for the most effective and clinically sound treatment goals.

---

### When integrating spirituality and art therapy:

- Be clear with clients about the orientation and scope of practice.

- Advise clients if physical touch is part of an integrated practice.

- Consider using a informed consent to outline practice parameters.

- Avoid dual relationships.

- Be aware of state and federal guidelines about healing touch (somatic) practices.

# References

## Introduction

American Art Therapy Association (2012) *American Art Therapy Association: Position Statement State Licensure for Art Therapists.* Available at www.americanarttherapyassociation.org/upload/2012policystatementstatelicensure.pdf, accessed on 12 February 2013.

American Art Therapy Association (2011) *Ethical principles for art therapists.* Available at www.americanarttherapyassociation.org/upload/ethicalprinciples.pdf, accessed on 9 January 2013.

Art Therapy Credentials Board (2011) *Code of Professional Practice.* Available at www.atcb.org/pdf/2011-ATCB-Code-of-Professional-Practice.pdf, accessed on 9 January 2013.

Corey, G., Schneider-Corey, M., and Callanan, P. (2007) *Issues and Ethics in the Helping Professions (8th ed.).* Belmont, CA: Thomson.

Green, A. R. (2012) "Ethical considerations in art therapy." *Canadian Art Therapy Association Journal 25,* 2, 16–21.

Hammond, L. and Gantt, L. (1998) "Using art in counselling: ethical considerations." *Journal of Counselling & Development 76,* 3, 271–277.

Henley, D. (2002) *Clayworks in art therapy: Playing the sacreal circle.* Philadelphia: Jessica Kingsley Publishers.

Hinz, L.D. (2011) "Embracing excellence: a positive approach to ethical decision making." *Art Therapy: Journal of the American Art Therapy Association 28,* 4, 185–188.

Kak, N., Berkhalter, B., and Cooper, M. (2001) *Measuring the competence of healthcare providers.* Quality Assurance Operations Research Paper from the Quality Assurance Project (USAID), 2, 1, 1–28.

Kapitan, L. (2011) "'But is it ethical?' articulating an art therapy ethos." *Art Therapy: Journal of the American Art Therapy Association 28,* 4, 150–151.

Kitzrow, M. A. (2002) "Survey of CACREP-accredited programs: training counselors to provide treatment for sexual abuse." *Counselor Education and Supervision 42,* 2, 107–118.

Koocher, G. P. and Keith-Spiegel, P. (2008) *Ethics in Psychology and the Mental Health Professions: Standards and Cases* (3rd ed.). New York: Oxford University Press.

Meara, N. M., Schmidt, L. D., and Day, J. D. (1996) "Principles and virtues: a foundation for ethical decisions, policies and character." *The Counseling Psychologist 24*, 1, 4–77.

Moon, B. L. (2006) *Ethical Issues in Art Therapy* (2nd ed.). Springfield, IL: Charles C. Thomas.

Newman, J. L., Gray, E. A., and Fuqua, D. R., (1996) "Beyond ethical decision making." *Consulting Psychology Journal: Practice and Research 48*, 4, 230–236.

Orr, P. (2012) "Technology use in art therapy practice: 2004 and 2011 comparison." *The Arts in Psychotherapy 39*, 4, 234.

Packard, T., Simon, N. P., and Vaughn, T J. (2006) "Board Certification by the American Board of Professional Psychology." In T. J. Vaughn (ed.) *Psychology Licensure and Certification: What Students Need to Know.* Washington, DC: American Psychological Association.

Pope, K. S., Sonne, J. L., and Greene, B. (2006) *What Therapists Don't Talk About and Why: Understanding Taboos That Hurt Us and Our Clients.* Washington, DC: American Psychological Association.

Pope, K. S., Tabachnick, B. G., and Keith-Spiegel, P. (1987) "Ethics of practice: the beliefs and behaviors of psychologists as therapists." *American Psychologist 42*, 11, 993–1006.

Prochaska, J.O., Norcross, J., and DiClemente, C. (1995) *Changing for Good: A Revolutionary Six-Stage Program for Overcoming Bad Habits and Moving Your Life Positively Forward.* New York, NY: William Morrow Paperbacks.

Trevino, L.K. and Brown, M. (2004) *Managing Organizational Deviance.* Thousand Oaks, CA: Sage Publications Inc.

Welfel, E. R. (2006) *Ethics in Counseling and Psychotherapy: Standards, Research, and Emerging Issues* (3rd ed.). Pacific Grove, CA: Brooks/Cole.

# Chapter 1

Amos, T. and Margison, F. (2006) "Fetters or freedom: dual relationships in counseling." *International Journal for the Advancement of Counseling 28*, 1, 57–69.

Behnke, S. (2006) "The discipline of ethics and the prohibition against becoming sexually involved with patients." *Monitor on Psychology 37*, 6, 86.

Blos, P. (1979) *The Adolescent Passage: Developmental Issues.* New York: International Universities Press.

Butler, S. and Zelen, S. L. (1977) "Sexual intimacies between therapists and patients." *Psychotherapy 14*, 2, 139–145.

Chesler, P. (2005) *Women and Madness* (2nd ed.). Hampshire, UK: Palgrave MacMillan.

Erikson, E. (1993) *Childhood and Society*. New York: W.W. Norton & Company Ltd.

Fisher, C. D. (2004) "Ethical issues in therapy: therapist self-disclosure of sexual feelings." *Ethics & Behavior 14*, 2, 105–121.

Jackson, S. and Scott, S. (2010) *Theorizing Sexuality (Theorizing Society)*. Maidenhead: Open University Press.

Kluft, R. P. (1989) "Treating the patient who has been sexually exploited by a previous therapist." *Psychiatric Clinics of North America 12*, 483–499.

Ladany, N., O'Brien, K. M., Hill, C. E., Melincoff, D. S., Knox, S., and Petersen, D. A. (1997) "Sexual attraction toward clients, use of supervision, and prior training: a qualitative study of predoctoral psychology interns." *Journal of Community Psychology 44*, 413–424.

Lamb, D. H. and Catanzaro, S. L. (1998) "Sexual and nonsexual boundary violations involving psychologists, clients, supervisees, and students: implications for professional practice." *Professional Psychology 29*, 5, 498–503.

Lamb, D. H., Catanzaro, S. J., and Moorman, A. S. (2003) "Psychologists reflect on their sexual relationships with clients, supervisees, and students: occurrence, impact, rationales and collegial intervention." *Professional Psychology 34*, 1, 102–107.

Masters, W. and Johnson, V. (1981) *Human Sexual Response*. London: Bantam.

Pope, K. S. (1990) "Therapist-patient sex as sex abuse: six scientific, professional, and practical dilemmas in addressing victimization and rehabilitation." *Professional Psychology 21*, 6, 227–239.

Pope, K. S. (1993) "Licensing disciplinary actions for psychologists who have been sexually involved with a client: some information about offenders." *Professional Psychology 24*, 3, 374–377.

Pope. K. S. (2001) "Sex Between Therapist and Client." In J. Worell (ed.) *Encyclopedia of Women and Gender: Sex Similarities and the Impact on Society and Gender* (vol. 2). New York: Academic Press.

Pope, K. S., Sonne, J. L., and Greene, B. (2006) *What Therapists Don't Talk About and Why: Understanding Taboos that Hurt Us and Our Clients*. Washington, DC: American Psychological Association.

Pope, K. S., Tabachnick, B. G., and Keith-Spiegel, P. (1986) "Sexual attraction to clients: the human therapist and the (sometimes) inhuman training system." *American Psychologist 41*, 2, 47–158.

Pope, K. S., Tabachnick, B. G., and Keith-Spiegel, P. (1987) "Ethics of practice: the beliefs and behaviors of psychologists as therapists." *American Psychologist 42*, 11, 993–1006.

Sonne, J.L. and Pope, K.S. (1991) "Treating victims of therapist-patient sexual involvement." *Psychotherapy 28*, 174–187.

Talwar, S. (2010) "An intersectional framework for race, class, gender, and sexuality in art therapy." *Art Therapy: Journal of the American Art Therapy Association 27*, 1, 11–17.

# Chapter 2

Allen, C.K., Earhart, C.A., and Blue, T. (1992) *Occupational Therapy Treatment Goals for the Physically and Cognitively Disabled.* Bethesda, MD: American Occupational Therapy Association.

Appelbaum, P. S. and Grisso, T. (1988) "Assessing patients' capacity to consent to treatment." *The New England Journal of Medicine 319*, 1635–1638.

Beattie, B.L. (2007) "Consent in Alzheimer's disease research: risk/benefit factors." *The Canadian Journal of Neurological Sciences 34*, 27–31.

Buchanan, A. (2004) "Mental capacity, legal competence and consent to treatment." *Journal of the Royal Society of Medicine 97*, 9, 415–420.

Budrys, V., Skullerud, K., Petroska, D., Lengveniene, J., and Kaubrys, G. (2007) "Dementia and art: neuronal intermediate filament inclusion disease and dissolution of artistic creativity." *European Neurology 57*, 3, 137–144.

Crutch, S.J., Isaacs, R., and Rossor, M.N. (2001) "Some workmen can blame their tools: artistic changes in an individual with Alzheimer's disease." *The Lancet 357*, 2129–2133.

Cruz de Souza, L., Volle, E., Bertoux, M., Czernecki, V., Funkiewiez, A., Allali, G., Leroy, B., Sarazin, M., Habert, M., Dubois, B., Kas, A., and Levy, R. (2010) "Poor creativity in frontotemporal dementia: a window into the neural bases of the creative mind." *Neuropsychologia 48*, 3733–3742.

Dastidar, J.G. and Odden, A. (2011) "How do I determine if my patient has decision-making capacity?" *The Hospitalist*, 24–31.

Deaver, S. P. (2011) "Research ethics: Institutional review board oversight of art therapy research." *Journal of the American Art Therapy Association 28*, 171–176.

Drago, V., Foster, P.S., Trifiletti, D., Fitzgerald, D.B., Kluger, B.M., Crucian, G.P., and Heilman, K.M. (2006). "What's inside the art? The influence of frontotemporal dementia in art production." *Neurology 67*, 1285–1287.

Finney, G.R. and Heilman, K.M. (2007) "Artwork before and after onset of progressive nonfluent aphasia." *Cognitive Behavioral Neurology 1*, 7–10.

Flaherty, A.W. (2005) "Frontotemporal and dopaminergic control of idea generation and creative drive." *Journal of Comparative Neurology 493*, 147–153.

Gordon, N. (2005) "Unexpected development of artistic talents." *Postgraduate Medicine 81*, 753–755.

Grisso, T., Appelbaum, P.S., and Hill-Fotoulu, C. (1997) "The MacCAT – T: a clinical tool to assess patients' capacitates to make treatment decisions." *Psychiatric Serv. 48*, 1415–1419.

Holmén, K., Ericsson, K., and Winblad, B. (2000) "Social and emotional loneliness among non-demented and demented elderly people." *Archives of Gerontology and Geriatrics 3*, 177–192.

Hunt, L.A. (2003) "Driving and dementia." *Generations 27*, 2, 34–38.

Karlawish, J. (2003) "Research involving cognitively impaired adults." *The New England Journal of Medicine 348*, 1389–1392.

Kim, S.Y.H. (2011) "The ethics of informed consent in Alzheimer disease research." *National Review Neurology 7*, 7, 410–414.

Kim, S.Y.H., Kim, H.M., Langa, K.M., Karlawish, J.H.T., Knopman, D.S., and Appelbaum, P.S. (2009) "Surrogate consent for dementia research: a national survey of older Americans." *Neurology 72*, 149–155.

Kim S.Y., Kim H.M., McCallum C., and Tariot P.N. (2005) "What do people at risk for Alzheimer's disease think about surrogate consent for research?" *Neurology 8*, 1395–1401.

Leo, R. J. (1999) "Competency and the capacity to make treatment decisions: a primer for primary care physicians." *Journal of Clinical Psychiatry 1*, 5, 131–142.

Love, C., Costillo, J., Welsh, R., Scott, S., and Brokaw, D. (2011) "Cognitive impairment and dangerous driving: a decision making model for the psychologist to balance confidentiality with safety." *Psychology 2*, 254–260.

Lowendfeld, V. and Brittain, W. L. (1987) *Creative and Mental Growth* (8th ed.). Upper Saddle River, NJ: Prentice Hall.

Malchiodi, M. (1998) *Understanding Children's Drawings.* New York: The Guilford Press.

Mell, J.C., Howard, S.M., and Miller, B.L. (2003) "Art and the brain: the influence of frontotemporal dementia on an accomplished artist." *Neurology 60*, 1707–1710.

Mendez, M.F. (2004). "Dementia as a window to the neurology of art." *Medical Hypothesis 63*, 1, 1–7.

Mendez, M.F. and Perryman, K.M. (2003) "Impairment of humanness in artist with temporal variant frontotemporal dementia." *Neurocase 9*, 42–49.

Miller, B.L., Ponton, M., Benson, D.F., Cummings, J.L., and Mena, I. (1996) "Enhanced artistic creativity with temporal lobe degeneration." *Lancet 348*, 1744–1745.

Miller, B.L., Cummings, J., Mishkin, F., Boone, K., Prince, F., Ponton, M., and Cotman, C. (1998) "Emergence of artistic talent in frontotemporal dementia." *Neurology 51*, 978–982.

Miller, B.L. and Hou, C.E. (2004) "Portraits of artists: emergence of artistic creativity in dementia." *Archives of Neurology 61*, 842–844.

Rankin, K.P., Liu, A.A., Howard, S., Slama, H., Hou, C.E., Shuster, K., and Miller, B.L. (2007) "A case-controlled study of altered visual art production in Alzheimer's and FTLD." *Cognitive Behavioral Neurology 20*, 48–61.

Rascovsky, K., Salmon, D.P., Lipton, M.D., Leverenz, J.B., DeCarli, C., Jagust, W.J., and Galasko, D. (2005) "Rate of progression differs in frontotemporal dementia and Alzhiemer disease." *Neurology 65*, 397–403.

Rascovsky, K., Hodges, J.R., Knopman, D., Mendez, M., Kramer, J.H., Neuhaus, J., and Miller, B.L. (2011) "Sensitivity of revised diagnostic criteria for the behavioral variant of frontotemporal dementia." *Brain 134*, 2456–2477.

Reisberg, B., Franssen, E.G., Souren, L.E.M., Auer, S.R., Akram, I., and Kenowsky, S. (2002) "Evidence and mechanisms of retrogenesis in Alzheimer's and other dementias: management and treatment." *American Journal of Alzheimer's Disease and other Dementias 17*, 4, 202–212.

Resnick, P.J. and Sorrentino, R. (2005) "Competence vs. capacity: an analysis for medical professionals. Forensic issues in consultation-liaison psychiatry." *Psychiatric Times 23*, 26–28.

Roberson, E.D., Hesse, J.H., Rose, K.D., Slama, H., Johnson, J.K., Yaffe, K., Forman, M.S., Miller, C.A., Trojanowski, J.Q., Kramer, J.H., and Miller, B.L. (2005) "Frontotemporal dementia progresses to death faster than Alzheimer disease." *Neurology 5*, 719–725.

Stallings, J.W. (2010) "Collage as a therapeutic modality for reminiscence in patients with dementia." *Art Therapy: Journal of the American Art Therapy Association 14*, 3, 136–140.

Stewart, E.G. (2004) "Art therapy and neuroscience blend: working with patients who have dementia." *Art Therapy: Journal of the American Art Therapy Association 21*, 3, 148–155.

U.S. Department of Health and Human Services: Child Welfare Information Gateway (2012) *Penalties for Failure to Report and False Reporting of Child Abuse and Neglect: Summary of State Laws.* Washington, DC: Child Welfare Information Gateway.

Vandenberghe, R. (2011) "Sense and sensitivity of novel criteria for frontotemporal dementia." *Brain 9*, 2450–2453.

# Chapter 3

Alders, A., Beck, L., Allen, P., and Mosinski, B. (2011) "Technology in art therapy: ethical challenges." *Art Therapy: Journal of the American Art Therapy Association 28*, 4, 165–170.

American Art Therapy Association (2011) *Ethical Principles for Art Therapists.* Available at www.americanarttherapyassociation.org/upload/ ethicalprinciples.pdf, accessed on 9 January 2013.

American Telemedicine Association (2009) *Practice Guidelines for Videoconferencing-based Telemental Health.* Available at www.atmeda.org/ files/public/standards/PracticeGuidelinesforVideoConferencing-Based%20 TelementalHealth.pdf, accessed on 9 January 2013.

Art Therapy Credentials Board (2011) *Code of Professional Practice.* Available at www.atcb.org/pdf/2011-ATCB-Code-of-Professional-Practice.pdf, accessed on 9 January 2013.

Brandoff, R. and Lombardi, R. (2012) "Miles apart: two art therapists' experience of distance supervision." *Art Therapy: Journal of the American Art Therapy Association 29*, 2, 93–96.

Haeseler, M. (1992) "Ethical considerations for the group therapist." *American Journal of Art Therapy 31*, 1, 2–9.

Hammond, L. and Gantt, L. (1998) "Using art in counseling: ethical considerations." *Journal of Counseling & Development 76*, 3, 271–277.

*Health Insurance Portability and Accountability Act of 1996* (1996) Pub. L. No. 104–191, 110 Stat. 1936.

Kapitan, L. (2007) "Will art therapy cross the digital culture divide?" *Art Therapy: Journal of the American Art Therapy Association 24*, 2, 50–51.

Moriya, D. (2006) "Ethical issues in school art therapy." *Art Therapy: Journal of the American Art Therapy Association 23*, 2, 59–65.

Orr, P. (2010) "Social Remixing: Art Therapy Media in the Digital Age." In C.H. Moon (ed.) *Materials and Media in Art Therapy.* New York: Routledge.

Orr, P. (2012) "Technology use in art therapy practice: 2004 and 2011 comparison." *The Arts in Psychotherapy 39*, 4, 234.

Porter, C. (2008) "De-identified data and third party data mining: the risk of re-identification of personal information." *University of Washington Shidler Journal of Law: Commerce & Technology 5*, 1, 3.

Silas, K. R. (2011) "The growing problem of camera phone abuse in health-care facilities." *Louisiana Bar Journal 59*, 3, 180–183.

Spaniol, S. (1994) "Confidentiality reexamined: negotiating use of art by clients." *American Journal of Art Therapy 32*, 3, 69–75.

## Chapter 4

Art Therapy Credentials Board (2011) *Code of Professional Practice*. Available at www.atcb.org/home/code, accessed on 7 May 2013.

Gerson, A. and Fox, D. (1999) "Boundary violations: The gray area." *The American Journal of Forensic Psychology 17*, 2, 57–61.

Henley, D. (2002) *Clayworks in Art Therapy: Plying the Sacred Circle*. London: Jessica Kingsley Publishers.

Herlihy, B. and Corey, G. (1997) *Boundary Issues in Counselling: Multiple Roles and Responsibilities*. Alexandria, VA: ACA Press.

Knapp, S.J. and VandeCreek, L.D. (2006) "Multiple Relationships and Professional Boundaries." In S.J. Knapp and L.D. VandeCreek (eds) *Practical Ethics for Psychologists: A Positive Approach*. Washington, DC: APA.

Knox, S. (2008) "Gifts in psychotherapy: practice review and recommendations." *Psychotherapy Theory, Research, Practice, Training 45*, 1, 103–110.

Koocher, G.P. and Keith-Spiegel, P. (1998) *Ethics in Psychology: Professional Standards and Cases*. New York: Oxford University Press.

Landgarten, H. (1981) *Clinical Art Therapy: A Comprehensive Guide*. New York: Brunner/Mazel.

Levin, S. and Wermer, H. (1966) "The significance of giving gifts to children in therapy." *Journal of the American Academy of Child Psychiatry 5*, 4, 630–652.

Malchiodi, C. (1998) *The Art Therapy Sourcebook*. Los Angeles, CA: Lowell House.

Pifalo, T. (2002) "Pulling out the thorns: art therapy with sexually abused children and adolescents." *Art Therapy: Journal of the American Art Therapy Association 19*, 1, 12–22.

Rutan, J. S. and Stone, W.N. (2001) *Psychodynamic Group Psychotherapy* (3rd ed.). New York: Guilford Press.

Spandler, H., Burman, E., Goldberg, G., Margison, F., and Amos, T. (2000) "'A double-edged sword': Understanding gifts in psychotherapy." *European Journal of Psychotherapy Counselling and Health 3*, 1, 77–101.

Stein, H. (1965) "The gift in therapy." *American Journal of Psychotherapy 19*, 3, 480–486.

Zur, O. (2007) *Boundaries in Psychotherapy: Ethical and Clinical Explorations*. Washington, DC: American Psychological Association.

# Chapter 5

Anderson, F.E. (1995) "Catharsis and empowerment through group claywork with incest survivors." *The Arts in Psychotherapy 22*, 5, 413–427.

Bartole, T. (2011) "Freud on touch: thinking sexuality in anthropology." *Esercizi Filosofici 6*, 376–387.

Burkholder, D., Toth, M., Feisthamel, K., and Britton, P. (2010) "Faculty and student curricular experiences of nonerotic touch in counseling." *Journal of Mental Health Counseling 32*, 2, 168.

Kearns, D. (2004) "Art therapy with a child experiencing sensory integration difficulty." *Journal of the American Art Therapy Association 21*, 2, 95–101.

Lowenberg, F. M., Dolgoff, R., and Harrington, D. (2004) *Ethical Decisions for Social Work Practice* (7th ed.). Belmont, CA: Brooks Cole.

Piaget, J. and Inhelder, B. (1969) *The Psychology of the Child*. New York: Basic Books.

Pope, K. S., Tabachnick, B. G., and Keith-Spiegel, P. (1987) "Ethics of practice: the beliefs and behaviors of psychologists as therapists." *American Psychologist 42*, 11, 993–1006.

Rubin, J. (2005) *Child Art Therapy*. Hoboken, NJ: John Wiley & Sons, Inc.

Sholt, M. and Gavron, T. (2006) "Therapeutic qualities of clay-work in art therapy and psychotherapy: a review." *Art Therapy: Journal of the American Art Therapy Association 23*, 2, 66–72.

Stenzel, C. L. and Rupert, P. A. (2004) "Psychologists' use of touch in individual psychotherapy." *Psychotherapy: Theory, Research, Practice, Training 41*, 3, 332–345.

Strozier, A.L., Krizek, C., and Sale, K. (2003) "Touch: its use in psychotherapy." *Journal of Social Work Practice 17*, 1, 49–62.

Swade, T., Bayne, R., and Horton, I. (2006) "Touch me never?" *Therapy Today 17*, 9, 41–42.

Zur, O. (2007a) *Boundaries in Psychotherapy: Ethical and Clinical Explorations*. Washington, DC: American Psychological Association Books.

Zur, O. (2007b) "Touch in therapy and the standard of care in psychotherapy and counseling: bringing clarity to illusive relationships." *U.S. Association of Body Psychotherapy Journal 6*, 2, 61–93.

## Chapter 6

Art Therapy Credentials Board (2011) *Code of Professional Practice.* Available at www.atcb.org/pdf/2011-ATCB-Code-of-Professional-Practice.pdf accessed on 9 January 2013.

Barnett, J. E. and Johnson, W.B. (2011) "Integrating spirituality and religion into psychotherapy: persistent dilemmas, ethical issues, and a proposed decision-making process." *Ethics & Behavior 21,* 2, 147–164.

Bolen, J.S. (1979) *The Tao of Psychology.* New York: Harper Collins.

Dein, S. (2004) "Working with patients with religious beliefs." *Journal of Continuing Professional Development 10,* 287–294.

Dow, J. (1986) "Universal aspects of symbolic healing: a theoretical synthesis." *American Anthropologist 88,* 1, 56–69.

Frame, M.W. (2000) "Spiritual and religious issues in counseling: ethical considerations." *The Family Journal 8,* 1, 72–74.

Furman, L. (2011) "Last breath: art therapy with a lung cancer patient facing imminent death." *Journal of the American Art Therapy Association 28,* 4, 177–180.

Gallup, G.J. and Jones, T. (2000) *The Next American Spirituality: Finding God in the Twenty-first Century.* Colorado Springs, CO: Victor.

Haldmen, D.G. (2002) "Gay rights, patient rights: the implications of sexual orientation conversion therapy." *Professional Psychology: Research and Practice 33,* 3, 260–264.

Hamdan, A. (2008) "Cognitive restructuring: an Islamic perspective." *Journal of Muslim Mental Health 3,* 1, 99–116.

Hodge, D.R. (2011) "Alcohol treatment and cognitive-behavior therapy: enhancing effectiveness by incorporating spirituality and religion." *Social Work 56,* 1, 21–31.

Kaufman, M.R. (1939) "Religious delusions in schizophrenia." *The International Journal of Psychoanalysis 20,* 363–376.

Kliewer, S. (2004) "Allowing spirituality into the healing process." *The Journal of Family Practice 53,* 8, 616–624.

Koepfer, S.R. (2000) "Drawing on the spirit: Embracing spirituality in pediatrics and pediatric art therapy." *Art Therapy Journal of American Art Therapy Association 17,* 3, 188–194.

Kubler-Ross, E. (1983) *On Children and Dying.* New York: Touchstone.

Lori, W. E., Blair, L.P., Gomez, J.H., McManus, R.J., Neinstedt, J.C., Serratelli, A.J., Vigneron, A.H., and Wuerl, D.W. (2009) *Guidelines for Evaluating Reiki as an Alternative Therapy.* Committee on Doctrine United States Conference of Catholic Bishops. Available at www.usccb.org/_cs_upload/8092_1.pdf, accessed on 3 February 2013.

Miller, W.R. (1998) "Researching the spiritual dimensions of alcohol and other drug problems." *Addiction 93*, 979–990.

Plante, T.G. (2007) "Integrating spirituality and psychotherapy: Ethical issues and principles to consider." *Journal of Clinical Psychology 63*, 9, 891–902.

Roberts, C. (2011) *Coping with Post-Traumatic Stress Disorder: A Guide for Families* (2nd ed.). McFarland & Company: Jefferson, North Carolina.

Sue, D. and Sue, D. (2008) *Counseling the Culturally Diverse: Theory and Practice* (5th ed.). Hoboken, NJ: John Wiley & Sons.

Suhail, K. and Ghauri, S. (2010) "Phenomenology of delusions and hallucinations in schizophrenia by religious convictions." *Mental Health, Religion & Culture 13*, 3, 245–259.

Swenson, J.E., Schneller, G.R., and Sanders, R.K. (2009) "Ethical issues in integrating Christian faith and psychotherapy: Beliefs and behaviors among CAPS members." *Journal of Psychology and Christianity 28*, 4, 302–314.

Tan, S. (2003) "Integrating spiritual direction into psychotherapy: ethical issues and guidelines." *Journal of Psychology 31*, 1, 14–23.

Tseng, W. and McDermott, J.F. (1981) *Culture, mind, & therapy: An Introduction to Cultural Psychiatry.* New York: Brunner/Mazel.

Van Hoecke, G. (2006) "Paradigms in Indian psychotherapy: applicability in a Western approach." *Mental Health, Religion & Culture 9*, 2, 119–125.

Zammit, C. (2001) "The art of healing: A journey through cancer: Implications for art therapy." *Art Therapy: Journal of the American Art Therapy Association 18*, 1, 27–36.

# Subject Index

# Author Index